HOW NOT
TO GET OLD

HOW NOT TO GET OLD

Jane Gordon

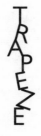

First published in Great Britain in 2020 by Trapeze,
an imprint of The Orion Publishing Group Ltd
Carmelite House, 50 Victoria Embankment,
London EC4Y 0DZ

An Hachette UK company

1 3 5 7 9 10 8 6 4 2

The moral right of Jane Gordon to be identified as
the author of this work has been asserted in accordance with
the Copyright, Designs and Patents Act of 1988.

A CIP catalogue record for this book is
available from the British Library.

ISBN (Hardback): 978 1 4091 9474 3
ISBN (ebook) 978 1 4091 9477 4
ISBN (Paperback): 978 1 4091 9475 0

Typeset by Born Group
Printed and bound in Great Britain by Clays Ltd, Elcograf S.p.A.

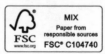

MIX
Paper from
responsible sources
FSC® C104740

www.orionbooks.co.uk

To the memory of my late mother,
the ageless Naomi Ryan, who was the inspiration
behind every single word in *How Not to Get Old*.

CONTENTS

HOPE I DIE BEFORE I GET OLD

For most of my life I have been blissfully in denial of the ageing process. Old age, I thought until quite recently, was something that happened to other people. It was never going to happen to *me*.

And it really didn't seem that it would. As I progressed through the decades, nothing much seemed to change. At forty I didn't feel any older than I had at thirty, at fifty I could still see my forty-year-old self in the mirror, and even at sixty — gulp — I didn't notice any obvious signs of the physical and mental decline that I associated with being *elderly*. Other people probably did, but they were kind enough not to say anything and as long as I stayed in my comfort zone — living in a cottage (that is probably a bit of a rut), surrounded by people of a similar age — I could convince myself I was in a permanent state of middle-agedness that would just go on and on.

There is no doubt I had luck on my side. I enjoyed, as they say, good health, rarely needing to seek medical help for anything more serious than a touch of flu or the odd infection.

I was lucky, too, in that my hair hadn't turned dramatically grey and my life had been so blessed that there were very few frown lines on my forehead. True, there were age spots on my hands, but since they had started appearing in my twenties I hardly noticed that they were filling out and multiplying.

And because I was still working as a journalist, I hadn't had to face the spectre of retirement. In the absence of any obvious changes to the way I lived my life, I was able to carry on in a blissful state of denial that time might one day catch up with me.

This was all pretty amazing, given that I had ignored most of the golden rules of a healthy lifestyle. Health and fitness weren't something I paid attention to. Even as a child, I wasn't what you might call sporty, and as an adult I had never managed to keep up a gym membership beyond its initial cut-price introductory month (usually giving up in the first week). And, no, I had never done yoga or Pilates or Zumba or whatever it is people do to tone and strengthen their bodies and relax their minds.

Moreover, the only diets that I had embarked on during my life had nothing to do with the *health* of my body, only the shape of it. The faddy diets of deprivation that I put myself through in my thirties in a bid to lose the elusive 'last seven pounds' of weight put on during three pregnancies should probably have impacted in some way on my sixty-year-old body — giving me high blood pressure or brittle bones — but, so far, they hadn't.

Of course I *knew* that switching to nutrient-rich foods would deliver sound physical benefits, but somehow I couldn't get enthusiastic about goji berries, quinoa or kefir, and I was never one of nature's vegans. Besides, if I was lucky enough to get away with eating a somewhat dubious diet of too many carbohydrates and too much salt and sugar without any obvious ill effects — type 2 Diabetes, high cholesterol or arthritis — there was no real incentive to change, so I didn't.

Even worse, my alcohol consumption consistently reached well above fourteen units a week. My defence for this particular excess was to claim that red wine — my 'poison' — was packed with antioxidants (not that I knew what the hell they were).

Nor, for that matter, had I done enough to support the sharpness of my brain — delegating the most taxing technological tasks to my adult children and refusing to embrace the kind of intellectual challenges that it needs if it is to maintain anything of its youthful speed and versatility. My grey matter was greyer than my still-quite-blonde hair.

But it wasn't the effects of alcohol, or poor dietary habits or even a lack of aerobic exercise that was the catalyst that forced me to stop and face the truth: that I was living a lie and was *not* — after all — immune to the ageing process.

What prompted this about-face was one of those events in life that you never see coming. I had not long turned sixty, and it was a rare perfect Saturday in an imperfect summer. At least, I think it was; I remember blue skies and the feeling — in the instant before it happened — that all was well in my world. Twenty minutes earlier I had picked up my son from the closest main-line station — ten miles away from my house — for a rare full-on family weekend.

After taking a back route through country lanes to avoid the usual Saturday traffic, we had just turned on to a short stretch of 60 mph dual carriageway half a mile from home when it happened. Our vehicle was hit by a driver attempting to overtake us before the road returned to one lane. The impact ricocheted our car from one side of the road to the other until we crashed sideways into a large signpost that brought us to a shuddering stop. The other driver, apparently unhurt, managed to pull up fifty yards or so further on.

What took place during and immediately after the moment of impact, in the clip of the accident that still makes me panic whenever I allow it to rerun in my brain, is something of a blur. I know that I thought — as did my son — that we were going to die. And I know too that it cannot have been very long before we established that we were both alive. I remember shouting, 'Are you all right?' and hearing my son saying the same words back to me over the sound of the car horn blaring on and on and on.

4

I remember, too, the enormous elation I felt when he got out of the car and stood beside me, repeating again and again, 'I'm OK, are you OK?' And at that moment I was OK — he was alive, I was alive and, despite the shattered state of the car and the splintered glass that I was covered in, there was hardly any blood.

It was only when I had been carried out of the car and was lying on the grass verge at the roadside that I felt anything other than relief. The pain arrived at the same time as the emergency services — the fire brigade, followed swiftly by a medic on a motorbike who gave me gas and air until the ambulance got there.

It was in hospital — suffering from nothing more serious than severe soft-tissue damage, a punctured lung and several hematomas (where an injury to the wall of a blood vessel causes blood to seep into the surrounding tissues) — that I was given a glimpse of what it would be like to be *old*. Unable even to sit up without the aid of two nurses, I discovered what it was like to be physically dependent on others — and I hated it. I felt helpless, vulnerable and lost.

In the course of a single difficult day I had gone from feeling immune to the ageing process to understanding what my life might be like in ten or twenty years when I would be officially *old*. As caring and gentle as the nurses and doctors were during that time I was relying on them to help me manage the most simple tasks, such as lifting me onto the bedpan; I felt stripped of my dignity, my independence and my sense of self.

Things weren't much better when I was discharged to the care of my family. Loving and attentive though they were, I found it difficult to accept that, without their help, I could not wash myself or make myself a cup of coffee. And although I did slowly begin to gain some of my former strength, I was unable to walk without crutches for several months and during that time became depressed and withdrawn. That car crash was rather like being visited by my own ghost of Christmases to come. How, I began to wonder, could I create a different future for myself? One in which I was mentally sharp and physically strong enough to remain independent and not become a burden on the NHS, my family and the state in my seventies, eighties and perhaps even nineties.

In the year or so following that near-death experience, I became aware of a growing desire to make changes to my life in an effort to achieve and maintain the physical and mental strength I needed to grow old in some form of grace. It wasn't just concern about becoming dependent on my three children (the law of averages making it possible that at least one of them will decide to whip me into a care home as soon as I show the slightest sign of senility) that played on my mind. It was the realisation that, unless I changed my ways, I might be unable to fulfil what I now believe to be one of the important roles and responsibilities of my life. To be a loving, inspiring, caring and, yes, sprightly grandparent to my granddaughter Edie and the grandchildren that are, as yet, twinkles in their parents' eyes.

6

These days, too, I am acutely aware of the ill health of others. I have entered that time of life when my contemporaries are falling prey to illnesses that break down their bodies and wear out their brains.

Of course, it isn't possible to eliminate the risk of developing a debilitating disease, but I know that I must safeguard against that eventuality.

* * *

So here I am, a clutch of years away from a milestone birthday I remain reluctant to admit, determined to do everything I can to . . . well, future-proof my mind and my body. Over the course of the year I will embark on a series of difficult challenges that will strengthen my chances of living long and strong.

I will research the tasks and programmes available, undertake the ones that seem best suited to me, and keep a record of my progress and the results. Ultimately, I want to get myself to a level of physical and mental fitness that will help me to move forward into a glorious, golden old age. Every part of my body from my core — via my temporal lobe — to my pelvic floor will be tightened, toned and strengthened.

Along the way there will be neuroscientists, gurus, dieticians, philosophers, poets, physicians, mad professors, tutors and personal trainers. With a little help, too, from my friends (chiefly my BFF Belle) and my family, I hope to go where no other woman 'of a certain age' has gone before to explore the ways it is possible to make the most of *later life*.

In taking on these challenges it is *not* my intention to chase the impossible dream of eternal youth (this book will be Botox-free) but to celebrate the joys of being 100 per cent *pro-* rather than *anti-*ageing.

So come with me on a journey that will, I hope, be as entertaining as it is informative, and learn — alongside me — How *Not* to Get Old.

1

STRICTLY BALLROOM

In which, even with two left feet, I learn to cha-cha-cha . . .

It's funny the way we can progress through life without ever acknowledging something that, deep down, we have known since we were children. Ever since I can remember, I've been a bit clumsy. As a small child, I found simple physical feats — like touching my toes — difficult. My idea of hell, from the age of six onwards, was school sports days. One year, partnered in the three-legged race (remember them?) with an equally uncoordinated member of my class, we fell over when the whistle blew for the 'off' and never got beyond the starting point.

Don't think for a minute that I'm about to complain of a hideous, unhappy childhood (I leave that to my children), because I had the perfect mother, a brilliant father, and I grew up feeling safe and protected, albeit a tiny bit bullied by my older, golden brother. While he was ridiculously athletic, hugely popular and in every school sports team, I was a sickly specimen who came last even in the sack race (you must remember them?).

By 'sickly' I mean that I suffered from bronchitis, which gained me at least a month off school every winter. And when I was perfectly well, I would claim to be ill to avoid things like playing netball, or hockey, going on cross-country runs, or vaulting the horse in gymnastics lessons. On one occasion, my mother rushed me to the GP's surgery after I complained of a bad stomach ache, and my performance of being in 'terrible pain' was so convincing that I found myself in the operating theatre of our local hospital having my healthy appendix removed.

Sporty, I wasn't. But my greatest failings were displayed in the compulsory ballet and country dancing classes at school, and later (in my teens) the ballroom dancing classes I attended at the Desdemona Bartlett School of Dance. By then I was hopelessly shy, clumsier than ever, and terrified at the very thought of learning to waltz in the arms of a strange, spotty boy who was probably as frightened of me as I was of him (back then all the schools in my area were single sex). I'm not sure why my parents put me through this particular ordeal; perhaps they had fantasies of my attending a coming-out ball and, like Cinderella, capturing the heart of a prince (or a duke or an earl or just someone very rich) after executing a perfect paso doble.

I can't remember how long I attended those weekly lessons before giving up. (I was that awful child who, having agreed to take something up — Sunday school, the Brownies, riding lessons, etc — would be whining to give it up within a fortnight.) And I never once used what I did or didn't learn (there was no coming-out ball or Cinderella moment).

In the intervening years, the only time I have ever enjoyed dancing, sadly, is when I am on my own and obsessed by a particular song that I put on repeat on my iPhone (and before that, on my Walkman). Usually this dancing would take place late at night in the kitchen after a glass or two of red wine when my children/husband/partner had gone to bed. During these solitary moments I could convince myself I had a hidden talent that, because of my shyness, I had been unable to develop.

In this, I was delusional. Had anyone happened to catch me dancing with myself, they would have laughed helplessly and told me I was terrible. This dreadful solo dance habit, which persists to this day, doubtless explains why I am single and have only ever had two boyfriends; it's widely accepted that if you can't dance you are probably not very good in bed (hips don't lie, and good dancers can keep perfect rhythm).

Anyway, this is a roundabout introduction to a challenge that I absolutely did not want to do. In fact, when I think about it, ballroom dancing classes top the list of activities I have no desire to engage in, ahead of jumping out of a plane at 13,000 feet, shark cage diving in South Africa or running with bulls in Spain. Because the truth is — as I should have known from that awful three-legged race — that I have *two left feet*.

But fate has a way of making us do the last thing we want to. And fate, in this case, takes the form of my BFF Belle, who turned up on my birthday with a small, beautifully wrapped present. I was excited because she has brilliant taste and a real gift for, well, gifts. I did my best to hide my disappointment at finding — when I ripped off the paper — a pair of shocking-pink leg warmers.

'How lovely,' I said with a fake smile.

'There's more,' Belle said. 'Look inside the card.'

'A ballroom dancing class?' I said, glancing in horror at the enclosed brochure.

'Yes,' she said. 'Eight till nine every Monday evening with this brilliant teacher — you must have seen him on *Strictly*. It's going to be *so* much fun . . .'

This was the first time in our five-year friendship that I had questioned whether Belle and I were singing — never mind dancing — to the same tune. Didn't she know me by now? Hadn't she picked up that I am not what you would call fleet of foot? And that if I didn't have a dog, the furthest I would walk on any given day would be the distance between my front door and my car? And who exactly was this person Ian Waite (our teacher) from this programme Belle loves but I have never actually watched?

* * *

In the two weeks leading up to our first lesson I watch endless YouTube clips of Ian Waite in his prime on *Strictly*

Come Dancing. It turns out he appeared in seven series of the show; his two most successful years were 2004, when he and athlete Denise Lewis were runners-up, and 2005, when he reached the final three with Zoe Ball.

These days (he's now forty-eight) he is still a celebrity with regular appearances on the *Strictly* spin-off show *It Takes Two*. Married to pilot Drew Merriman (their wedding was splashed across at least eight pages of *Hello!* magazine), he not only teaches ballroom but has also created a dance exercise programme called FitSteps, 'featuring all your favourite *Strictly* dances' in a forty-five-minute aerobic session that is available across the UK. On his website I discover that for £35 I can get a poster-sized autographed photograph of Ian still looking as dashing as he did fifteen years ago.

The more I research him, the more nervous I am. So I try to come up with reasons why (apart from my two left feet) I can't attend the Beginners Ballroom class that Belle so *generously* bought me for my birthday.

What finally forces me to give in is the discovery that dozens of studies across the world indicate that ballroom dancing classes offer huge benefits to older adults. And this fits perfectly with the premise of this book.

A 2010 report released by the Centre for Policy on Ageing (CPA), 'Shall We Dance', reviewed international evidence on the health benefits of dancing as we age. The study reveals that 'dance has been shown to be beneficial in the direct treatment of a number of conditions including arthritis, Parkinson's disease, dementia and depression'. It also claims that taking part in ballroom dancing reduces the chances of developing dementia by 76 per cent (it is, apparently, far more difficult to learn than it looks and acts as an aid to both the brain and the body of older students).

If this isn't enough to prove that these classes will be one more way for me to future-proof myself against a dramatic decline in my physical, mental and cognitive skills, a Swedish research programme cited in the 'Shall We Dance' report offers further encouragement. They followed two groups of older people — one group were regular amateur dancers while the other had no history of dancing or sporting activity. They discovered that, as they aged, the dancers showed 'superior performance in reaction times, motor behaviour and tactile and cognitive performance'. The study concluded that the far-reaching beneficial effects in the dancing group 'make dance, beyond its ability to facilitate balance and posture, a prime candidate for the preservation of everyday life competences of elderly people'.

In addition, ballroom dancing is inclusive. Anyone and everyone can take part (even me), and of all exercise-based classes it has the lowest drop-out rate. Which, hopefully, will mean that after a fortnight of ballroom dancing, I won't be whining to Belle that I want to give up (unlike my childhood self).

As this is the first time, probably since I left school, that I have taken an exercise class, and it is my first physical challenge in my attempt not to get old, I am a little worried about the dress code. Will I have to wear a typically *Strictly* costume — something garishly coloured and covered with feathers, glitter and sequins? And what about the shoes? I have a paltry selection of high heels and they are all black (no gold, silver or scarlet). I glance at images on Google and decide that I have nothing in my wardrobe that is vaguely suitable, although I do have an ancient white evening gown that looks very Tess Daly.

When I call Belle to ask what she will be wearing, she tells me not to be ridiculous and wear my 'gym gear' and trainers — and to bring a water bottle because it says on the website we will need to hydrate. I don't own any gym wear, and am not invested in the idea of dancing enough to actually go out and buy some. Instead, I find an old pair of tracksuit bottoms at the back of my wardrobe and match them with a much-worn white T-shirt and the pair of New Balance trainers that my younger daughter left in my house some months ago.

It goes without saying that when I pick up Belle — several years my junior and not just my best friend but also my best-dressed friend — on that first Monday she is wearing head-to-toe colour-coordinated Lululemon dance/gym wear. Her trainers are top of the range and she is carrying a water bottle she found on Net-a-Porter that contains healing crystals (mine was lent to me by my granddaughter and is bright pink and covered in cartoon kittens).

When we arrive at the venue (a school hall in Wokingham) there is already a long queue waiting to be let in. Looking around, I feel a little less jittery. For a start, Belle and I are by no means the oldest of the beginners; nor are we, from the ratio of women to men, going to be the only female same-sex couple. As we wait, it suddenly occurs to me that perhaps Belle would rather be here with her husband instead of an unfit woman with two left feet.

'Oh no,' Belle assures me. 'Ed won the British Junior Latin Championship at Blackpool in 1966. That's another reason for coming with you; I could never compete with him.'

We all file in — most people pay on the door, but Belle has prepaid for the whole term for both of us — and take our place on the floor. There are, I reckon, about fifty beginners, around a third of whom are singles.

Belle and I already knew that in ballroom dancing old-fashioned gender roles are strictly adhered to, so one of us would have to be the 'man' and one of us would be the 'woman'. Since Belle is 5' 8" in her bare feet (and about 5' 10" in her fancy trainers), and I am probably now about 5' 4" (although I swear I was 5' 6" before I had children), it is logical that she should take the 'male role'.

It is at this point, while all the singles are attempting to couple up, that we get our first glimpse of our teacher. He's 6' 3", lean and absurdly elegant. With the added glamour of his dancing celebrity, Ian Waite in the flesh (with his shirt famously half unbuttoned to reveal his six-pack) is awesome. Maybe he has gone a little too far with the fake tan (Belle insists he has probably not long returned from a break in Barbados), but the way his sun- (or bottle-) kissed skin brings out his brilliant blue eyes is stunning to behold. When he smiles — and boy, does Ian Waite smile — his perfect white teeth, strip-lit by the harsh ceiling lights, positively sparkle.

In an instant we are all — even me, but particularly Belle — in thrall to him.

We are to start, he informs us, with the basic steps of the waltz. This is so easy, he says, that 'a child of three could learn'. I am instantly worried that someone at the other end of the age spectrum — me, for instance — will not find it so simple.

'It's a smooth, gliding dance in three-four time with a familiar one, two, three rhythm,' Ian tells us. Already I am lost.

He divides us into the two gender groups — the men and the women — because, although the steps are the same, the order in which we take them differs. Belle joins seven other women in the 'men' group, who (as historically men have always done) 'take the lead' in the dance while the women merely 'follow'.

To the count of one, two, three, Ian teaches Belle's group to put their 'left foot forward, right foot to the side and close, reverse, right foot back, left foot side and close'. As I watch Ian and the 'men' go through their paces, somewhere at the back of my brain something pings and I remember learning these steps at Desdemona Bartlett's School of Dance. This, I think, is going to be fine. What on earth was I worried about?

But then it's time for Ian to teach the women. It turns out that we, as nature's followers, start by moving our right foot *back*, left foot to the side and close. This is perfectly simple when Ian teaches us on our own, but it gets complicated when Belle and I put our arms in the correct male/female position and try to do the basic box step together. For some reason I can't keep pace with Belle and find myself consistently putting the wrong foot forward.

'No,' Belle says again and again as I repeatedly get it wrong. 'You start with your right foot back, not your left foot forward, *do you see*?'

But I don't see. While the other beginners are now in sync with each other and managing a few steps, I am struggling.

'You know I find it hard going backwards,' I whimper.

It gets worse when Ian informs us that — since we can't just move in one direction — we have to learn how to turn. Worse still, we are going to do this with *music*. Obviously, there isn't room here for the *Strictly Come Dancing* Band, so Ian has recordings for the various dances which echo round the hall via a speaker system that is so loud even the oldest beginners can hear.

Then we have to learn how to reverse turn to the stirring sound of Vera Lynn's 'Anniversary Waltz'. I try, I really try, but all that backwards movement that the follower (i.e. the female) has to do is too difficult for someone with my lack of spatial awareness. Belle mutters that dancing with me is like going on the bumper cars at the fair, because as we move we keep accidentally banging into other couples going the other way. This at least makes me laugh, which nothing else does (I'm close to tears several times before the hour is up).

It's clear that Ian has picked us out as one of the problem couples. He comes over to help, but even with a *Strictly* professional as my 'leader', I can't work out which leg should be going which way. Then he takes Belle — in the female role — for a spin; despite having occupied the male role so far, she looks almost as professional as Motsi Mabuse.

He then suggests that Belle and I swap roles so that I am the man and she is the woman, on the basis that this will allow me to go forwards (as the leader) more than I have to go backwards. Men's steps, I discover, are simpler than the woman's to allow for the fact that they have to lead.

'But I can hardly lead my dog,' I mutter.

'That's because you never trained him,' Belle bites back.

With practice, we realise Ian is right: I find being the man far easier than being the woman.

By the end of our first lesson, with Belle simultaneously following, leading and stopping to explain what I am doing wrong, I am exhausted and she is beginning to regret her birthday gift — albeit not quite as much as I am.

The next morning Belle sends me a WhatsApp message saying she is already feeling a 'bit toned'. She adds that she is 'fine with our sexual transition', because clearly I am happier 'presenting as a man'. My reply is simple: 'I really DO have two left feet' (with an emoji of a bare foot). Belle messages me back to point out that the emoji I sent was a *right* foot.

In preparation for Week 2 (the cha-cha) Belle keeps sending me links to YouTube videos in which a series of professional teachers and their partners demonstrate how easy it is for a beginner to learn the cha-cha. This is another 'simple' dance with a basic step done to the rhythm 'one, two, cha-cha-cha'.

Belle also sends me backup clips of scary teachers and their partners demonstrating the basic box step of the waltz, so I can 'practise at home every evening'. I find time every night to do half an hour's practice, gliding myself romantically round my living room to the sound of Simply Red singing 'If You Don't Know Me by Now' and Norah Jones' classic, 'Come Away With Me'.

As a result of my hard work — and fear of Belle's fury — I have managed to remember all the steps from last week. Repetition, it would seem, is the key to adult learning. And when Ian, as dazzling as ever, starts us off on a recap of the waltz he taught us last week, even Belle is impressed by my footwork.

That done, Ian separates us into our gender groups (which means that this time I am with the boys) to teach us the basic steps of the cha-cha ('step, replace, cha-cha-cha, step, step, cha-cha-cha').

In Week 2 a little inter-couple bonding is starting to take place. I have linked up with a young man called Dave who is due to marry his fiancée Emma — who has bonded with Belle. Emma has persuaded him to take the classes so that they will be able to perform a perfect first dance at their wedding (something that I thought was very twentieth century but is, according to Belle, having a bit of a comeback).

Dave and I, at least on the dance floor, have a lot in common. Neither of us is here by choice and we share a tendency to put the wrong foot forward (or back). While Ian teaches Belle and the female group the woman's steps (which are more or less the same), Dave and I attempt to repeat what we have just learned, saying the steps out loud (which, I am to discover in several other challenges, is an effective way to help me remember what I am trying to learn). The other men (and the women taking the male role) look at us rather contemptuously. We realise, as the weeks go by, that the male leader group are more openly competitive than the female followers (no surprise there, then).

When Belle and I come together to practise the cha-cha steps as a couple, we are quite good. This is mostly because the 'hold' is looser with some space between us and it's almost impossible not to get in the rhythm when the music playing is Sam Cooke's 'Everybody Loves to Cha Cha Cha'.

It's fast and fun, unlike the waltz, and when we manage to learn the crossover break (AKA New Yorks — check them out on YouTube) — Dave and Emma applaud us.

A little while later the music changes to a contemporary track — Camila Cabello's 'Havana' — and I find that, against all the odds, I am enjoying myself. I am beginning to see why dance can become addictive. It's early days, but when you find yourself 'in step' with your partner (which from time to time I do) it feels wonderful.

At home that night I download 'Havana' and find myself singing it out loud and happily doing a solo version of the cha-cha all round my house.

Belle sends me a message the following morning saying, 'Weren't we fab last night! I think we may be cracking it.' Fingers crossed, I am beginning to believe that she is right.

It turns out we are both a little overconfident. When we turn up for Week 3, in place of the lovely Ian (who is away filming) we have his father, Alan, who is a lot tougher (and shorter) than his glamorous son. He informs us that he plans to teach us two dances this evening — the quickstep and the social foxtrot — and my heart sinks.

The quickstep, he tells us, is a 'light-hearted dance that is fast and powerfully flowing'. This sends Dave and me (as we learn the man's move) into a panic. We are taught the chasse — side-together-side — and that's OK, but we have problems with the 'reverse turn' and the 'forward lock', never mind the 'fishtail' (there are so many strange terms for the turns and twists you do in ballroom that only add to the difficulty of learning, let alone remembering, the steps).

Belle's woman's group, I notice when it's their turn to learn their moves, are much more relaxed and bonded than the men. Dave and I are the only two who openly admit our difficulties and attempt to encourage each other.

When we are all put together to practise with our partners, it's immediately clear that yet again I am going to let Belle down. The music doesn't help as it's the song from Disney's *Jungle Book*, 'I Wanna Be Like You'. I am trying so hard to be quick that I trip over Belle's foot and go flying into the wall. Alan gets one of his female assistants to take Belle's place and help me, but since that doesn't make much difference he tells me to 'practice at home' as it's time to move on to the next dance.

'The social foxtrot,' Alan declares as he begins to explain the movements, 'is an easy-to-learn step for beginners. The kind of dance that can make you look as if you know what you are doing when you take to the floor on your cruise this year.'

While Belle and I have no intention of taking a cruise together (although she does suggest that I might benefit from one of those Saga ship trips for over-sixty singles), we are excited by the idea of a dance that really is 'simple'. And simple it is, with its basic 'forward with the left, forward with the right and slide close right foot to left' movement. Dave and I rehearse while Alan teaches the women's moves and we are amazed to discover we have almost mastered the steps.

'Do you think Emma and I could do the social foxtrot for our first dance at the wedding?' he asks me and I just nod, aware, when the sound of 'Let's Face the Music and Dance' comes over the loudspeaker that, easy as it seems, he might not be, well, Fred Astaire to Emma's Ginger Rogers.

Belle and I are almost perfectly in sync with this dance and we end the lesson feeling so positive (despite my poor quickstep) that she suddenly announces she is going to buy a proper pair of dance shoes and a dress for next week. I think this is linked to the fact that Belle has become a vegan and the combination of our exhaustive new routines and her diet has resulted in a loosening up of her Lululemon leggings (not that they were ever tight).

As we leave, Alan stops me to tell me that I am the kind of pupil 'who will have forgotten the steps by the time I get to the car park' and that practice, practice, practice is the only way I will be able to retain all the information I take in each week. I feel quite offended that he has singled me out for this advice — he says nothing to Dave — but I know he is right. I have become aware that — doubtless because I am at least twenty-five years older than Dave — I will have to work harder to keep up.

* * *

On Week 5 (Week 4 is cancelled because the school is closed for half term) Belle and I arrive feeling pretty good about our progress. We have practised and practised (alone and together) almost every day since Week 3. Besides, Belle is wearing what she describes as a 'purple chiffon leotard dress with a flared asymmetric skirt' that she insists she bought for 'just over £10' on Amazon, and a pair of silver, open-toed, ankle-strap, high-heeled ballroom dancing shoes that she claims were £4.99. She had offered to get me a black men's mesh Latin dance shirt but I declined and instead put on a white shirt, velvet jeans and a pair of black patent brogues I already had in my wardrobe (I have always liked mannish clothes).

A lot of the beginners have made a similar effort — although Belle is the only one in purple — and there is a real sense of camaraderie developing. Learning a new skill in a multi-generational group, I have discovered, is interesting and rather uplifting. The youngest of us is only seventeen and the oldest in their eighties, with just about every age in between. And as we progress there is a kind of breaking down of the barriers that so often restricts one generation from bonding and socialising with another.

This feeling of oneness with people younger and older than Belle and me is an unexpected bonus of the lessons, as I had assumed that ballroom dancing was very much a senior activity. In reality, primarily due to the success of *Strictly Come Dancing*, it now has much wider appeal.

Ian is back from filming and at his glamorous best, and since we had lost a week he decided to just recap on what we had learned so far, which is a huge relief.

Dave and I are still struggling with the fishtail move in the quickstep (which involves stepping outside your partner and then crossing so you are standing between their legs).

In Week 6 we add the jive to our repertoire and Belle is so good that Ian uses her to demonstrate exactly how the dance should be done. And although I feel a pang of resentment that she is clearly teacher's pet, at least it leaves me free to hide at the back of the class (just like at school, this is my go-to place). As a result, I don't get very far with the jive (but neither does Dave).

By now, though, I am gaining confidence in several of the other dances, particularly the cha-cha and the simple social foxtrot. I've noticed, too, that I am more energetic, fitter and — maybe for the first time in my life — I feel as if I am properly inhabiting my own body and taking control of my movements. I am also feeling positive about life in general. This may be linked to taking on something I didn't *want* to do but have done anyway (thanks to Belle), and discovering that, while I am by no means brilliant (still struggling with the quickstep), I am doing OK and experiencing a welcome sense of accomplishment.

In Week 7 we move on to the American smooth, which is a composite dance using steps from the waltz, the Viennese waltz and the foxtrot. Again, Ian chooses Belle as his partner to demonstrate the moves. Of course, she performs perfectly in the arms of her hero, but it doesn't go so well when she is back with me.

I long ago realised that there is probably nothing physical that Belle can't do better than me (she is naturally athletic). And while I am happy with what I have managed to learn over the last couple of months (next week is the final lesson of the term) and have enjoyed the classes *so* much more than I expected, I can't help but feel that I have held her back.

At the end of Week 8 — when it is time to say goodbye — Belle and I have mixed feelings. We are sad to be parting from Dave and Emma — who *are* going to do the social foxtrot at their wedding because the steps are a perfect match for 'their' song, 'The Way You Look Tonight' — but we are reluctant to book for next term. Although we feel we have benefited mentally and physically from the discipline of ballroom dancing, we don't want to go any further. I can't imagine where I would ever use these new skills and, as good as she is, Belle still doesn't think she will be a match for her husband, Ed (who has two shelves in his study packed with the dancing medals and trophies he won in his youth).

Yet we don't want to give up the routine we have got into of regular Monday dance classes, so instead we enrol in Ian's spin-off exercise class, FitSteps. This is aerobic and fun but still uses the steps we've learned in ballroom. That way I'll continue to flex my cognitive muscles in remembering the movements, while building up strength in my hips so that I might be able to dance my way into my seventies and eighties (without, I hope, the need to have them surgically replaced).

* * *

My favourite FitSteps routine (we go every week) remains the cha-cha, when Ian plays 'Havana'. Even now, as I write this, the song is playing (*Havana, na-na-na*) in my head and my feet are involuntarily starting to move. And do you know what? I now have just *one* left foot which, would you believe, is perfectly in sync with my right . . .

2

SACRÉ BLEU!

In which I attempt to become bilingual . . .

I am sitting in Professor Jon Simons' office in the Behavioural and Clinical Neuroscience Institute at Cambridge University, talking through the things I might do to improve my cognitive skills in my bid *not* to get *old*.

Among the ideas he puts forward are one or two that he deems 'essential' if I am to make any real progress in stimulating my brain. And the first of these is the *command* that I take up a new language. Not just any language, either. Ideally it should be one that uses a different alphabet or system of symbols.

'Mandarin would be ideal,' Professor Jon comments as I nervously skim through his A – Z of possible languages, 'because it's the hardest language to learn and the most widely spoken native language in the world.'

I look blankly at him and he sighs.

'If that's going to be too tough, you could perhaps try something simpler. Greek, for instance,' he continues.

'In three months — which is all the time I've got before I go on holiday?' I squeal. 'I'm one of those people who have to go through the whole English alphabet to remember that Q comes before R. How am I going to cope with the Greek alphabet?'

Professor Jon, who is young (well, about forty) and handsome and *so* clever that he probably speaks a dozen languages, is bemused to learn that I can only speak one.

'Surely you did Latin at school?' he asks.

I shake my head.

'French?' he fires back.

'Well, I did get a CSE in French back in the days when you took CSEs if you weren't likely to pass a full-on GCE,' I say.

'Can you remember any French?' he asks.

I think for a moment and then come up with the few words and phrases that have somehow lodged in my brain.

'La plume de ma tente! S'il vous plaît! Je ne comprends pas! Merci! Sacré bleu!' Zut alors!' I manage to roll out.

'You know what?' Professor Jon says in quite excited tones. 'Relearning French could be even better for your brain than Mandarin, because it will jog your long-term memory and sharpen your short-term memory.'

He goes on to explain that when we start to talk as small children we do so by absorbing the language, or languages, we hear in the background of our life. The older we get, the more difficult learning a new language becomes, and as a result it is cognitively very beneficial for the brain. In working our brains harder, we are exercising them. This is believed to increase our neuroplasticity, altering the brain structurally and functionally by creating new connections that help it to keep running flexibly and efficiently as we age.

'Which is exactly what you need,' Professor Simons concludes.

In the 1980s researchers discovered that some individuals who, while alive, had showed no obvious symptoms of dementia, were at autopsy found to have undergone changes to the brain that indicated advanced Alzheimer's disease. It was thought that the reason these people did not exhibit dementia symptoms was because they had built up what scientists term 'cognitive reserve' during their lives. Their brains had been stimulated by a lifetime of education and curiosity which helped them to offset the damage and to continue to function as usual.

Ongoing research by Dr Thomas Bak at the School of Philosophy, Psychology and Language Sciences at the University of Edinburgh suggests that even short-term learning of a new language can help us maintain our mental agility. In 2016 Dr Bak led a study which assessed the attention levels of a group of students aged eighteen to seventy-eight before and after they attended a one-week course in Gaelic. The results were then compared with those of students who had attended a one-week course that didn't involve learning a language; while both groups showed improvement, the Gaelic learners' performance was significantly better.

'I think there are three important messages from our study. Firstly, it is never too late to start a novel mental activity such as learning a new language. Secondly, even a short intensive course can show beneficial effects on some cognitive functions. Thirdly, this effect can be maintained through practice,' Dr Bak stated when the study was published.

Professor Simons is slightly sceptical about such studies and suggests that at my age learning French in three months (let alone one week) will involve a great deal of hard work. Although there are various low-cost ways of learning languages online, in his opinion I will need one-to-one tutoring because taking in so much new information in such a short time will require 'very effective teaching'.

* * *

On the drive back from Cambridge I am feeling a little anxious. My experience of French teachers has been far from positive. I have chilling memories of being humiliated as a child by the sadistic Mademoiselle Dupont, and on parents' evening with my two daughters I was as terrified as they were of their teacher, known simply as *Madame*.

Then in a flash of inspiration I remember my friend Arnaud Barge, who happens to be the author of a series of French textbooks and a renowned personal tutor.

I got to know Arnaud and his partner Gareth through mutual friends, and we regularly get together for a game of Scrabble (Arnaud, incidentally, can play Scrabble in six languages — and win). He agrees to take me on and seems confident that by the time I am due to go on my family holiday — in France — I will be ready to do 'all the talking'.

At this point Arnaud had no idea how little I remembered from my long-lost school days. I was the kind of pupil who always rushed for the back row no matter what the subject (except perhaps English) and spent most of my French lessons doodling in my exercise book or staring out of the window. I can't claim any learning disorder (dyslexia, ADHD, etc), though I was — as my mother liked to put it — *a late developer*. My real problem was sheer laziness.

Still, I was brimming with optimism (another of my lifelong failings) when I arrived at Arnaud's house for my first lesson. Arnaud, I should probably mention, is young, handsome, beautifully dressed and full of Gallic charm. An accomplished chef, he runs his private tutoring business — which he calls Arnaud's Language Kitchen — from the kitchen of his home.

There are, he tells me, 100,000 words in the average French dictionary, but today Arnaud simply wants to gauge how many I can remember. To that end he has assembled a collection of common kitchen items that I am supposed to identify as best I can in French.

'Have a look at the objects I have selected and — from your long-term memory — see how many you can name with reasonable accuracy. Don't worry about pronunciation, spelling, grammar or anything like that for now,' he tells me.

I study the twenty-eight items — all of which I can easily identify in English — for about ten minutes as I attempt to retrieve the corresponding word in French. For heaven's sake, surely I know the words for cup, saucer, fork, plate and spoon? But the only immediately recognisable object is *une télévision* a word which, Arnaud informs me later, is a cognate, i.e. the same in English and French (usually because the word is derived from Latin). I struggle on for a while and manage to come up with *une assiette* (a plate), and a few almost-cognates (*une serviette* — a napkin; *une spatule* – a spatula; and *un livre* – a book). With a few heavy hints from Arnaud — whom it emerges is the absolute antithesis of the fearful old Mademoiselle Dupont — I eventually succeed in identifying six of the twenty-eight simple words he expected me to recall.

'*Sacré bleu*, Arnaud!' I say despairingly. 'I know nothing!'

'You will certainly be exposed as knowing nothing if you ever say "*Sacré bleu!*" in France,' Arnaud scolds. 'Or that other English idea of a French blasphemy, "*Zut alors!*" They are expressions that these days are only used in the headlines of British newspapers whenever they report a French news item. They are old-fashioned, and no longer in common use. The equivalent British phrases that a French newspaper might use would be "Golly gosh!" or "Gadzooks!" Tell me honestly, when did you last hear those expressions when you were shopping in Sainsbury's?' Arnaud continues before moving on to the next stage of our lesson. I am suitably chastised.

'OK, now my question is,' he says in his hopeful voice, 'why have I divided these twenty-eight items into two groups – one set closer to you and one set closer to me. And that, actually, is a bit of a clue.'

Then it comes back to me – the total horror of the fact that everything in French is, as I put it to Arnaud, male or female.

'Well done!' he exclaims. 'Rule number one in French is that absolutely everything has a gender.'

For the rest of the lesson Arnaud gives me the French words for all twenty-eight items. Through a series of simple tests, and a lot of repetition (I already know from my ballroom dancing classes that for older learners you need an awful lot of repetition to retain anything in your brain), I manage to identify them all. Then he does something cruel: he times how long it takes me to list the words in French. I manage it in just over five minutes.

I drive home feeling overconfident and full of enthusiasm for the homework Arnaud has set me from the textbook he deemed most appropriate for my abilities. It's called *Talk French for Rusty Learners*. In three months, he tells me, I should be able to move on to *Talk French for Confident Speakers*. Fingers crossed.

The first homework exercise seems simple enough. All I have to do is decide which of the twenty French nouns is masculine and which is feminine. Thankfully, the words are all singular. During our lesson, I have grasped that most feminine nouns end in *e* or *ette* or *eille*, so it only takes me three hours (and the backup of my French dictionary) to get it right.

'*Bonne, bonne*,' Arnaud praises me when he marks my work, and I have to admit I glow at this. If I was overconfident at the end of Lesson 1, I am ridiculously cocky (*le coq* m., *la poule* f.) at the start of Lesson 2. In fact, I am so sure this challenge is going to be, well, easy-peasy, that my inner feminist (the strident one) emerges and I berate Arnaud (as if it's *his* fault) about the gender bias in the French language.

'Explain to me, please, Arnaud,' I say, 'why is masculine always the default setting in French?'

'I'm afraid that's just the way it is,' he replies. 'Even foreign words imported into French are masculine — *le tennis, un weekend*, and so on. The only foreign word I can think of that is feminine is *une pizza*.'

'You mean in France it really is a case of "*cherchez la femme*"!' I say, thrilled by my first — albeit rather feeble — attempt at a bilingual joke.

But I don't stop there. I go on, and on.

'Why, Arnaud,' I continue, 'is my fork a girl and my knife a boy? Is there any possibility that the feminine *chaise* I am sitting on could present itself as masculine? Is there anything in French that can be *non-binary*?'

We spend (or should I say 'waste') the rest of the lesson debating whether France is a man's world, at least so far as French-language purists are concerned.

Arnaud concedes that linguistically there is opposition in modern-day France not just from the LGBTQ+ lobby but also from French feminists who are irate about the fact that all professions (with two exceptions: nurse *une infirmière* and maid *une femme de chambre*) are masculine.

In Lesson 3, Week 3, we tackle when to use *être* (to be) and when to use *avoir* (to have) in relation to different verbs and physical descriptions.

Finally something sounds a bell from my schooldays. Mademoiselle Dupont forced us to learn *être* by rote on pain of death (is there any English person over the age of, say, forty who can't recite *je suis, tu es, il est, elle est, nous sommes, vous êtes, ils sont, elles sont*)?

But I had no recall of the fact that 'to be' (*être*) is used when you are describing someone's height, weight and general character. Nor did I remember that 'to have' (*avoir*) is used when referring to someone's age, hair and eyes. Arnaud then gives me a list of English sentences that I have to translate into French using either 'to be' or 'to have'.

The first two sentences I find quite easy to translate and not a little flattering.

Je suis grande et j'ai les cheveux longs et blonds et les yeux bleus: 'I am tall and have long blond hair and blue eyes'. (I am 5' 4" with shoulder-length greying-blond hair and grey eyes — I told you Arnaud had a lot of Gallic charm.)

The second sentence is even more over the top: *Je suis drôle et intelligente. Je suis mince et j'ai les cheveux raides*: 'I am funny and clever, I am thin and have straight hair'. (I am not thin and, although I try to disguise it, I have curly hair. I leave it to you to judge if I am, er, *drôle*).

* * *

I could go on to describe, in minute detail, each of my lessons with Arnaud for the entire thirteen weeks, but it would probably bore you as much — sadly — as it began to bore me. Which isn't to say that I didn't enjoy my hour-long sessions with Arnaud — I loved them. It wasn't the work we did together that I found tedious, it was my inability to remember what I had learned the previous week and the laborious homework I had to complete.

Homework always was a problem for me (I believe that these days some schools have banned it because of the unnecessary stress it puts on both pupils and teachers, not to mention parents!). Having homework at my age — and remember I am simultaneously trying to learn a dozen other things that are meant to be sharpening me up, physically and mentally — is even worse than it used to be. The experience has dragged me back to those terrible years at my convent school (before I was asked to leave) when I was always in the bottom five in the class, and my excuses for not doing my homework were beyond ridiculous.

My excuses are still pretty unbelievable. I turned up in Arnaud's Language Kitchen in Week 7 and told him

Le chien a mangé mes devoirs (the dog ate my homework). Zorro, my dog, didn't of course (his thing is socks) and I could tell from Arnaud's weary expression that he didn't believe me.

To my credit, I did attempt to boost my progress by buying — on Arnaud's advice — some 'simple' French children's books. I found a copy of the French version of *Where's Wally?* (*Où est Charlie?*) on eBay. But it didn't improve my reading skills, because looking for Charlie — who, not surprisingly, wears the same bobble hat, glasses and red-and-white striped jumper as our English Wally — doesn't involve many words.

Then I had the bright idea to go on Amazon and order a handful of Roger Hargreaves' Mr Men and Little Miss books in French. Curiously, it turns out that, although the default setting in French is always masculine, there seems to be a great deal more sexual equality in the lives of children.

Little Miss Chatterbox, for example, translates to *Madame Bavarde* (Mrs Talkative) in the French edition. (There are no 'little misses' in France, just monsieurs and madames.) And while I enjoyed reading the six I ordered, and positively delighted in Mr Greedy's transformation into *Monsieur Glouton* (Mr Glutton) and Mr Bump's reincarnation as *Monsieur Malchance* (Mr Unlucky), my favourite — and the one that made my six-year-old granddaughter laugh the loudest at — was *Madame Oui* (Little Miss Yes). The one thing I learned from this particular exercise was that it was going to take me a lot longer than three months to reach the stage where I could read Flaubert's classic *Madame Bovary* in the original French.

Next, also on Arnaud's advice, I downloaded an audiobook for children entitled *10 Bed-Time Stories in French and English*, written and narrated by Frédéric Bibard. For several weeks I was lulled to sleep every night by Frédéric's seductive voice on my iPhone, and I think I did pick up a smattering of conversational French from listening to his stories. But I have to admit I was more interested in the man than anything he was saying (in French or English). I found myself googling him and developing a crush.

* * *

Curiously, my Week 9 lesson — numbers and dates — goes really, really well. Which comes as a surprise because I struggle with numbers and dates in English; maths was probably the weakest of my weak subjects in my schooldays. Yet, reaching into my long-term memory, I discover that I can count from *un* (one) to *cent* (one hundred) without thinking. Arnaud, who is beginning to panic as we move closer to my final few weeks of lessons, breaks into applause when I recite my numbers fluently. He then asks me to tell him the only six numbers in the French language that contain the word '*et*' (and).

I think he is going to faint when I reply, '*Vingt-et-un, trente-et-un, quarante-et-un, cinquante-et-un, soixante-et-un, soixante-et-onze.*'

With two weeks to go before my planned family holiday in Toulouse — which will be the real test of how much French I have learned — Arnaud is worried that, while I certainly have progressed, I have not given enough time to the subject. I defend myself by reminding him that I have so many other brain-boosting tasks going on that I am finding it difficult to distinguish between a double clef (my music lessons) and a *double entendre*.

For our last two sessions, we decide I will focus on mastering a couple of dozen expressions that I am likely to need in Toulouse. Thankfully, I'm not going on a French exchange where I would be living with a local family and talking in French all the time. I will be staying with my own English-speaking family, and only conversing in French when I am shopping, ordering in a restaurant or asking directions.

'What you need to comfortably get under your belt are the expressions that you will use most in France. The things you want to buy, the places you want to go, the things you urgently need — transactional language. In these situations, you won't have to say long complicated sentences. If you overdo it and use complex French, it will result in the person you are talking to assuming you are fully fluent and he or she will talk back to you in a vocabulary that you are not yet able to cope with. Then you will be lost. It will be white noise,' Arnaud tells me.

He concentrates on teaching me basic phrases; simple verb and noun combinations that I can use in almost any tourist scenario.

'Don't think for hours, rehearsing in your head what you are going to say to the person selling cheese at the market. Point at what you want and say *Je voudrais* (I would like) and then say *combien* (how much), using what I call the "antipodean inflection", where you raise your voice at the end of any statement or sentence to turn it into a question.'

As subtly as I can — bearing in mind that Arnaud is French — I voice my concern that his fellow countrymen do not always seem receptive to my countrymen. It's probably a myth, or at any rate an overdone stereotype, but a lot of British people believe that the French do not like them. Consequently, they can seem quite rude when, for instance, you are trying to buy cheese from them at a market.

'You need to use polite little phrases as stepping stones,' he reassured me. 'Just use your *Je voudrais* (I would like) plus a verb such as *aller* (to go) and then add wherever it is you want to go — *à la piscine* (to the pool), for example, or *en ville* (to town) — and you're done. Behave just as you would if you were buying something or asking someone a question in Britain; if you use positive body language, lots of smiles and *merci* and *s'il vous plaît*, you will be fine. Minding your P's and Q's and smiling will never go amiss in any country, especially France,' he concludes.

At our final lesson he gives me more stepping-stone phrases that, if I can lodge them in my brain, I will be able to use again and again. *Je vais* (I am going), *le prendre* (I'll take it — as in the cheese or whatever) and *J'ai besoin de* or *d'* (I need) used for anything from *un taxi* to *un timbre* (a stamp).

Arnaud reminds me, as Professor Jon had done at the outset, that I will have to work hard to remember these shortcut French phrases. Making the connections that help us memorise things gets increasingly difficult as we grow older and the brain becomes set in its ways. 'A baby is not born programmed to speak Greek or Latvian, they speak what they are exposed to when their brains are growing and malleable.'

I point out that babies with their fresh young brains take about eighteen months to grasp the words for mummy, daddy and dog, while I've managed to get beyond that in only three months *at my age*. Arnaud laughs and gives me some typed-out sheets of useful stepping-stone phrases, and I feel quite emotional as I tuck them and my now worn copy of *Talk French for Rusty Learners* under my arm and prepare to leave Arnaud. How will I cope without him next week when I am buying cheese at the market in the medieval village of Lauzerte?

As we part, I thank him and say I hope I will be OK, but I realise in order to be fully fluent I will need to return for the autumn term.

'After all, Arnaud, it's not as if I'm off to France to discuss Brexit with President Macron,' I jest.

'Not yet, anyway. But when I am finished with you next term — maybe,' is his response.

Nous verrons! (We'll see!)

* * *

It is exactly three months since I was sitting in Professor Jon's office deciding which language I should try to learn, and here I am — in a café in the historic market square in Lauzerte, plucking up the courage to order food and drink for my family. I remind myself that it was my intention to do 'all the talking' on this holiday. How difficult can it be? My daughter Bryony wants a black coffee and a croissant, my son-in-law Harry (who is a pretty fluent French speaker) would like a brioche and a glass of orange juice, and my granddaughter Edie, six, is insistent on having both a hot chocolate and a *pain au chocolat*. Everything we want is on the menu (complete with accompanying English translation, despite most of the words being — as Arnaud has taught me — English and French cognates). Besides, the waitress who comes to our table couldn't be more welcoming, so what can possibly go wrong?

'*Je voudrais avoir*,' I cautiously begin, before pausing to work out what comes next, '*un café noir, un croissant, une brioche, un jus d'orange, un chocolat chaud et un pain au chocolat*.'

It has taken me a full three minutes to get up the nerve to say this perfectly simple sentence. When I've finished, the waitress patiently says, 'And for yourself?' in predictably perfect English.

'Oh, I'll just have a cappuccino,' I mutter, fully aware that Bryony, Harry and Edie are struggling to stifle their laughter.

'I think I might be better in a supermarket, don't you, Harry? Because you don't have to say much apart from *combien* and *merci beaucoup* at the checkout,' I say, making light of my first far-from-fluent attempt to speak French. Trying to get all the words in the right order to form a sentence in French reminds me of that memory game we used to play when my children were small: 'My aunt went to Paris . . .'

'Yes, we can drive to the big Intermarché tomorrow morning,' Harry replies in a kind way (because he is very kind).

If there is one thing I love to do when I am, well, *abroad*, it is to go supermarket shopping, especially at those huge ones that have in-store pharmacies and bakeries. I don't know what it is about it that appeals to me so much, because it isn't as if I'm similarly excited by a trip to my local Tesco, but pushing my trolley (after having located a euro and put it in the right place) round the aisles of Intermarché with Edie at my side was probably the highlight of my holiday.

Edie, of course, is at the age where she is still confident that her Annie (the name she has called me since she first tried to say the word granny) knows more than she does. And as we wander round the store I find myself showing off to her, pointing out some of the things that I can recall the French word for: '*Pastèques!*' (watermelons), '*Pommes de terre!*' (potatoes). Edie, however, is anxious to get to the *jouets* (toys). She wants to buy an inflatable *licorne* (unicorn) and an *énorme pistolet à eau* (enormous water pistol) for the pool back at the villa, and who am I to deny my precious granddaughter anything that she wants?

Except, perhaps, the thing she spots in a *réservoir d'eau* (tank of water) on the *comptoir à poisson* (fish counter).

'Annie, Annie!' she cries. 'I want a crab! I can take it home and it can be my pet!'

There are about twenty furious-looking crabs in the tank, and as Edie attempts to pick one out, the man behind the counter asks, '*Puis-je vous aider*?' ('Can I help you?') I manage to reply '*Merci, je me fais que regarder*' ('Thank you, I'm just looking') before dragging a reluctant Edie away from *les crabes*.

By this time our trolley – or rather, *chariot* – is full to the brim with all manner of wonderful things. Now comes what I'm hoping will be the *pièce de résistance* of our shopping trip – the checkout or, as it is known here, *la caisse*. Because I am anxious to impress Harry – who has also filled a shopping trolley full of goods (mostly *le vin*) and is behind me in the queue – I have pre-prepared what I am going to say to the checkout person (something Arnaud absolutely bans, insisting that you speak French in 'the now').

When Edie and I have unloaded our *chariot* and the *caissière* (checkout person) has finished ringing everything up, I get ready to deliver my well-rehearsed lines.

'*Bonjour, mademoiselle*,' I begin. '*Comment allez-vous? Excusez-moi, puis-je payer en espèces ou par carte de crédit?*' (which, I am pretty sure, means something like 'Good morning, miss. How are you? Excuse me but can I pay in cash or with a credit card?')

The young woman has an expression on her face that is very similar to that of the women at the checkout of my local Tesco on particularly busy Saturday mornings. She is tired, she probably won't finish her shift till 9 p.m. and she is not remotely interested in whatever this madwoman behind this particular chariot is trying to say. I had been expecting her to chat to me a little, perhaps returning my pleasantries, bidding me good morning and asking how I am.

But instead she responds — at the speed of lightning — in a language I don't recognise (it might as well be Mandarin or Greek to me):

'*Vous avez des sacs? On a aussi une promo sur les jouets de piscine; deux achetés, un troisième gratuit. Vous en avez besoin d'un troisième,*' she says, and I am lost. It is, as Arnaud warned me, 'white noise'.

To my relief, Harry steps forward to interpret. It seems French supermarkets do that same three-for-two-thing as their British counterparts. The problem is, our free water toy is in an aisle at the furthest end of the store and it takes Edie a full five minutes — once we get there — to settle on a pair of pink goggles (*lunettes de natation*).

When we make it back to *la casse* it isn't just the *caissière* who has an irritated look on her face; the shoppers queuing behind Harry are glaring at me in the way I would glare at them if the situation was reversed. As I hurriedly put my card in the *lecteur* (reader) and punch in my pin number, the *caissière* looks up and says, '*Avez-vous la carte de fidélité??*'

This time, miraculously, I understand what she is asking me: have I got a loyalty card?

'*Non*,' I reply with a smile although it would probably be worthy applying for one, because I will be back here next summer and, as I said, there is nothing I love more than supermarket shopping *quand je suis en France.*

* * *

Back home in the not very *Royaume-Uni* (United Kingdom) I am feeling better for my time in the sun, but nervous about the two calls I have to make to report on the progress of my *Français challenge en France.*

The first is to Arnaud, who inevitably answers the phone with a jaunty, '*Bonjour, ça va?*' (Hello, how are you?)

'*Ça va*,' I respond '*Ça va?*'

'*Ça va*,' he replies, before getting to the point (the French can have whole conversations consisting of asking each other how they are).

'*Comment ça s'est passé?*' Arnaud finally asks (which I think means 'How did it go?')

'*Comme ci comme ça! Au secours! J'ai besoin de* more lessons' I answer, which translates to something along the lines of, 'So-so! Help! I need more lessons'.

Having booked in for another ten lessons, I then make the call to Professor Simons, to update him on how my frontal lobe held up in France.

The only plus to this conversation is that we have it in English. Clearly, the Prof is disappointed that I am not yet fluent in French.

'I did warn you that it would involve working very, very hard to achieve fluency in another language in three months,' he says, implying that I didn't put in enough work (which obviously I didn't).

But he is heartened to hear that I have committed to further tuition, and encourages me to put in more time and practice because (as I already understand) repetition *is* key for the older learner.

'At your age it takes longer to lodge information in the brain and less time for it to fall out of your memory after it gets there. So keep going, Jane. And stay focused, because the better your French gets, the better your brain will be working,' he says as he ends the call and I get back to work.

À suivre . . . (To be continued . . .)

3

ROAD BLOCK

In which I attempt to become an advanced driver
(and finally learn to parallel park) . . .

Of all the challenges I am embarking on in my exhaustive attempt to take control of the ageing process, trying to pass the Institute of Advanced Motorists (IAM) test is probably the most daunting. But the idea of finding myself in a situation where I might have my licence taken away, or, as is currently being mooted, facing a retest when I hit seventy, make it an essential part of my, er, journey.

Since I don't live in a city in which it might be possible to get around on foot or public transport (the nearest bus stop to my home is a two-mile walk away and the buses run just once an hour), my car is almost as important to my quality of life as the roof over my head.

My car accident woke me up to why road safety might be of paramount importance in more ways than one. In the 60 mph collision, not only did I find myself facing the reality of my own mortality, in the aftermath I also came to realise how vital driving was to my independence. In the six-week or so period that I was on crutches, even walking to the nearest supermarket was impossible.

Moreover, since my car was a write-off and Harvey Keitel was unable to visit me in hospital with keys to a brand-new car (you must remember him reprising his *Pulp Fiction* role of Winston Wolfe in those insurance ads?), I had a foretaste of what life would be like without motor mobility (it took over three months for all the paperwork to be completed). Kind and caring though it was for my neighbour to suggest I sign up for the community bus service into town (for which he was a volunteer driver), it made me feel, far too early in life, like a charity case. The one time I did book a seat on the once-weekly minibus, I felt as if I had aged at least twenty years in two months (the other passengers were in their eighties), and the experience only added to my depression and fear of what might happen on the road ahead.

Besides, if I am honest, I have never been that confident behind the steering wheel. Indeed, one of the luckiest aspects of that collision was the fact that I was *not* driving the car. Thankfully, my son, who is an exemplary driver and had held a clean licence for eight years, was in control that day and it was his skill that prevented us from suffering greater damage (his own injury being whiplash, treated and quickly cured with physio and ibuprofen).

When I look back on the early years of my motoring life I sometimes wonder if I should ever have passed my test at all. My first test was a fail before it even started: I pulled out of a side street on to a main road and into the path of an oncoming car. Thankfully the driver of that car had the sense to emergency-brake so that a dramatic collision was avoided (although there was a slight dent to my side-mirror and a much bigger one to my dignity). I did pass on my second attempt, but I came away with a limited driving licence: I found gears so complicated, I opted to take the automatic-only test.

One of my most vivid driving memories is of that first magical night when it was legal for me to drive my husband's car on my own without anyone bossing me from the passenger seat. After I had put the children to bed (Bryony, then four, and Naomi, then two) and served up dinner, Jack (my then husband) graciously gave me the keys to his black convertible Golf and I set off for the M4 (ten minutes away).

The sense of liberation I felt when I hit 70 mph on the motorway was overwhelming; at that moment, the radio began to blare out the Eurythmics' 'Love is a Stranger' ('Love is a stranger in an open car/to tempt you in/and drive you far away'). It was as if the song had been written for me – I *was* the stranger in the open car, I *was* Annie Lennox. Of course I wasn't that fabulous slender, cropped-blonde, 1980s pop goddess; I was a slightly plump, somewhat matronly stay-at-home mum. But for a few mad minutes it was as if I had no responsibilities and that I could go wherever I wanted – all the way to the last junction on the motorway and beyond. In the end, I came to my senses and exited at Junction 7 (Slough) and, slightly deflated, drove back to Junction 1 and the family home in Chiswick.

While I did manage to complete that particular journey without incident, the early days of my driving life were not without a few . . . er, scrapes. My sense of spatial awareness has never been great; looking back, I think the real reason neither of my daughters have shown any interest in learning to drive is because of the childhood trauma of being strapped into the back of my car when I hit something — most often a tree or a kerb, but from time to time a parked car.

Bryony insists I once backed into a brick wall that dramatically collapsed, but I have no recall of this incident. Naomi remembers another time when, allegedly, I drove the wrong way up a busy one-way street.

* * *

The first car that I had to myself was a top-of-the-range second-hand Volvo estate that my husband bought at a bargain price from a slightly dodgy business associate. And while it did indeed have a state-of-the-art stereo system (for its time) and heated seats (unheard of then), there was something very wrong with its engine, which would overheat in dense traffic. Eventually (after several near-death moments in London) it caught fire on a trip the girls and I took to Devon (we came home by train, the Volvo is probably still on the A38).

In 1989 what had started out as a hobby (writing Boy George/George Michael fanzines from home) became a career and I was given a column on the now-deceased *Today* newspaper. My 'women's interest' opinion page on Wednesdays (a slot on all the nationals that *Private Eye* termed 'Glenda Slag') was headlined 'Jane Gordon at the Heart of Today'. I was giddy with excitement with this new role and as I was now earning more than pin money, I bought my own car: a cream Peugeot 208 that I drove with my (by now) customary abandon.

A colleague at the time, who has remained a friend, recalls a list of terrible mishaps that occurred while she was in the passenger seat. Jane Moore (yes, a Loose Woman) swears that I once drove over a pedestrian's foot, that I reversed into a parking pole, and that there was so much clutter in the passenger seat foot-well — including what she describes as a 'mountain' of parking tickets — that she had to sit with her knees up near her chin.

Indeed, the unpaid parking tickets very nearly gave me a criminal record when one day a police officer arrived at my home prepared to arrest me if I didn't pay my outstanding debts (I promptly did).

I could go on recounting my motoring misdeeds but the real point of this chapter is to tell you about my adventures with Des, the Chief Observer for my area of the Institute of Advanced Motorists. Our first meeting — set up during a brief phone call — took place at the unlikely-sounding Dobbies Garden Centre, where Des suggested we could park our cars and have an introductory coffee.

There is a lot of talk these days about women (in particular) suffering from *imposter syndrome*, which is the inability to believe in your skills or achievements. Sitting down opposite Des — easily identified by his IAM fleece and briefcase — I was overwhelmed with the feeling that I didn't deserve to be here. I was a *terrible* driver, what was I thinking of, embarking on an advanced driving course? Too often, Belle has to park my car when we go on an expedition together.

What made this sense of unworthiness worse — although I have no intention of telling Des unless I have to — was the fact that I had taken the free online DVLA Theory test earlier that morning. Most of the questions seemed ridiculously easy (almost infantile) e.g. 'You are travelling along a motorway and you feel tired, where should you stop to rest? a) On the hard shoulder? b) On a slip road? c) At the nearest service area or d) On the central reservation?' Or 'What should you do if you leave your car unattended for a few minutes? a) Leave your engine running? b) Switch engine off but leave keys in? c) Park near a traffic warden? d) Turn off the engine and lock the car?'

To my horror, when I pressed the result button it flashed up FAIL. I had only 38 of the 50 correct. This *proves* I am a charlatan because, of course, like anyone who took the driving test before 1996, there was no theory involved. Answering one or two simple questions from the examiner was the only proof you needed that you had opened your copy of the Highway Code. If there had been a theory test back in 1984 (yes, that long ago!) it would probably have taken me six or seven attempts to get on the road.

Still, I can't back out now, so I nervously explain to Des the premise of my book and why I need his help to ensure that I can drive safely into the future.

I doubt there is anyone on the planet better informed than Des about the rights and wrongs of driving and the statistics on collisions.

'In the Thames Valley, the average age of drivers in fatal collisions is fifty-one. We tend to think it would be younger than that because injuries from road accidents are the leading cause of death among people aged fifteen and twenty-nine,' he tells me over coffee.

The reason the average is so high, he explains, is because older people pick up bad habits, drive on automatic (rarely properly concentrating), and often go too slowly which can be as hazardous as speeding. I am doing the right thing, he tells me with an encouraging smile, in enrolling on a course that will help me to become a more confident and roadworthy driver.

'Although your driving licence officially runs out when you are seventy, you can renew it every three years thereafter by simply declaring you are fit to drive. At present, you don't have to take another test. For some older drivers it may be forty or fifty years since they took their original test, and it was a very different world back then. The big question is when do you give up your keys? Because no one wants to give up their independence,' he adds.

He goes on to tell me that these days the police no longer talk of road traffic *accidents* because, according to Des (and of course Freud), there is no such thing. Of what they now term *collisions*, 92 per cent are caused by human error — nine out of ten times someone is at fault.

'This course,' Des continues, 'is as much about unlearning as learning, identifying the bad habits you have developed and just focusing on driving. Driving is one of the most dangerous things we ever undertake and yet what we tend to do when we get in a car is think about everything other than driving. You might be thinking about the argument you had with your partner, what you are going to cook this evening and whether you are going to be late. Life has become more complicated and as a result we are trying to do too much, multitasking and always in a hurry, which impacts on our driving capability.'

This idea, that the last thing we are thinking about when we are driving is what we are actually doing, sets off a red light in my brain. How often — particularly on journeys I take regularly — have I found myself so absorbed in my thoughts or something on the radio — that I am driving on autopilot. Already, and we haven't got in a car yet, I am glad I have found Des.

Before I am allowed to get behind the wheel, Des is going to give me a demonstration of what passing the test and becoming an official Member of the Institute of Advanced Motorists (with a certificate, a chrome enamel car badge to put on your front grille and, hopefully, lower car insurance) involves.

This starts with an external 'visual inspection' to check that the vehicle maintenance is up to date; that the tyres are fully inflated and the wing mirrors are in position (and so on). Members are expected to carry out these pre-drive checks every time they start their car for the first time each day. And it doesn't end there; once we have opened the doors and entered Des's car, he explains that advanced drivers conduct an exhaustive 'cockpit drill'. In the manual it's stressed that this is something we should do automatically, in the same way 'we would expect an airline pilot to run through a series of pre-flight checks'.

When Des finally starts the engine and demonstrates a 'moving brake' test (essential before you move off), I am seriously thinking of opening the passenger door and running for the hills. Except, of course, I know that Des — who has two sons — will undoubtedly have a child lock to keep me (and his boys) from escaping.

Des's driving is faultless, as you would expect from a Chief Observer who — to date — has *never* had a pupil fail the advanced test (so no pressure there, then). I am recording his 'spoken thoughts' on my iPhone. This is where the driver — looking ahead and using a system called IPSGA (Information, Position, Speed, Gear, Acceleration) — narrates aloud every road sign, change in speed limit and potential hazard that might impact on 'the progress of the journey'. Journey, obviously, has a double meaning here because I am literally and physically embarking on a journey into the unknown (the A4 between Maidenhead and Reading).

'I am up to fifty but there are brake lights ahead,' Des says. 'Blue behind me, black to my side.' We refer to other cars as colours, not makes of car. 'Now silver has pulled in front of me, there are pedestrians offside and a cyclist ahead. White emerging from a concealed entrance presents a danger on the left so I am moving into what we call a zone of relative safety.'

Des's 'spoken thoughts' continue all the way back to the Dobbies car park, when it will be my turn to drive Des along the same route. I get off to a bad start because I have driven my mini straight into the parking space, instead of reversing in 'as all advanced drivers would'. Des informs me that I will have to learn to do this as a matter of course at all times (even in the Saturday rush hour at Tesco when only the quick and cunning forward-parker gets a space). This concerns me because one of the things I haven't revealed to him yet is that I have a problem moving *backwards*, especially in a car.

Still using what Des calls the 'creep-and-peep method', I manage to reverse out of the space. Before you can say Lewis Hamilton, I am roaring down the A4 at — Des informs me — 10 mph above the 40 mph speed limit. I slow down as he explains that becoming an advanced driver isn't about moving faster, it is about being able to move smoothly and safely from one limit to another. On the whole, Des seems reasonably safe in the passenger seat of my car (I don't notice him flinch once) and the only negative thing he has to say is about my habit of over-indicating, which I tend to do even if there isn't another car in sight.

Back in the car park, Des gives me an encouraging pep talk.

'You made a good start Jane,' he tells me. 'Without question, refreshing your driving is the best thing you can do to protect yourself as you get older. Even the most competent drivers can lose confidence, they might feel intimidated driving in a big city or they might become fearful of driving at night, and eventually they stop driving altogether. When we have finished this course, that won't be happening to you for a long, long time.'

Des then takes my IAM Course Logbook and gives me marks on the various 'competency levels' listed. A score of 1 is 'Commended', 2 is 'Satisfactory' and 3 'Requires development'. I am commended in only one of the thirty-four graded columns: I get a 1 for my eyesight. Everything else is 3, apart from 'courtesy to other drivers' and 'vehicle sympathy' (whatever that means), both of which win me a 2. If I am to pass the test, I will need at least a 2 in every one of the thirty-four columns, including 'slow manoeuvring' — the IAM term for parallel parking (reversing!). As optimistic as Des is, I can't help feeling that I have taken on an impossible challenge.

ROAD BLOCK

In the comment box, Des lists the various things I need to work on and sets me 'homework'. This week it is to use 'spoken thoughts', talking aloud to myself when I am driving anywhere in the next few days. I am not, he says, allowed to listen to the radio or one of my audiobooks as this can disturb my concentration, which is vital when 'everything hangs around this concept of the thinking driver'.

As it happens, the following day I have to drive to Bexhill to visit a sick relative. This isn't an easy journey as it involves the M4, M40, M25, the A21 and the A2690 (I could go on, but I don't want to lose your attention). Anyway, it's a dull, grey, wet and windy day and Zorro the dog and I set off from home at dawn expecting to reach our final destination at noon. (Several weeks later, it turns out to be the final destination of my sick relative too.)

When Zorro is in the passenger seat I tend to talk to him even though I am fully aware that he has a rather limited vocabulary. Most days he only responds when I say 'squirrel', 'good boy', 'supper' or 'Catty' (he has a hate-hate relationship with my fourteen-year-old cat). And although I like to think he tries to understand when I talk to him about more complex subjects (politics, the meaning of life, and so on) he is easily bored.

But on this particular 'spoken thoughts' day I am expected to continue this one-sided conversation for the entire journey. To my surprise, I quickly realise that this is a clever way of ensuring that I keep my eyes on the road, and sometimes a little ahead of it (which is pretty much what advanced driving is all about). Zorro is confused by my stream-of-consciousness, and since nothing I say is of interest (no squirrels in the road, etc.) he dozes off.

So far our progress has been smooth, but when we hit the M25 Google Maps informs me that there is an hour-long queue ahead due to an accident, 'but you are still on the fastest route'. Once through the jam I carry on speaking my thoughts but give up about twenty minutes from my destination when Google Maps begins speaking over me (it's a wriggly route). By this time I have almost lost my voice. I forgive myself because it's early days − it takes about five months for the average applicant to be ready for the test − and with my history it could take a lot longer.

In Lesson 2, back in Dobbies car park, Des tells me that as well as being a Chief Observer for IAM he is a 'blood-biker', working through the night once a weekend delivering emergency blood for the NHS. Since both of these worthy endeavours are voluntary, I begin to wonder about Des's day job. I have a hunch he might be a senior policeman (he is very tall and authoritative), but since he is also very patient and encouraging it's possible he's a social worker of some kind. Then it turns out that he has a PhD in Philosophy and is a university lecturer. This, as you can imagine, makes me even more nervous and eager to please. Des, frankly, is a bit of a legend.

This second session is chiefly about teaching me something Des ironically calls OAP (Observation, Anticipation, Planning), particularly when it comes to roundabouts. The one rule I do stick to at roundabouts is giving priority to drivers on your right. But I am often in the wrong lane and I am also wrong to stop at a roundabout when I can see there are no other cars in my way. The golden rule is that you should 'plan to stop but look to go'.

Des has dozens and dozens of little expressions and the one he repeats most today is 'believe what you see'. At the end of the lesson when he marks my competency levels in my Advanced Driver Course Logbook I fear that I am (figuratively) going backwards rather than forwards. But when I get home I see that I have achieved six grade 2s ('Satisfactory') although written in capital letters is the instruction HIGHER LEVELS OF CONCENTRATION REQUIRED.

It's Lesson 3 and, since time is short (and these sessions can sometimes take two and a half hours), Des directs me to a road that leads to an industrial complex where we can practise my braking skills. We do emergency brakes (great fun), and soft brakes, and Des reveals that the best drivers rarely use their brakes at all because they have mastered IPSGA. One of the worst driving sins, according to Des, is driving on your brakes, not only does it result in a bumpy journey, it makes life very difficult for the drivers behind you.

At the end of the lesson Des has given me seven grade 2s and four grade 1s. I am commended for my rolling brake test, my approach to vulnerable road users (I successfully overtook a cyclist), my general road courtesy and eyesight (the one unchanging mark throughout my course). I drive home feeling just a little superior to the other motorists on the road.

At some point in our fourth lesson Des decides that it would be a good idea if I could observe one of the most common driving errors that people make. We drive to a narrow country road and park, hidden from the vision of passing motorists, close to a blind bend. This is perhaps one of the most bizarre exercises I undertake with Des, because he directs us behind a tree so that neither we or our parked car can be seen from the road. Peeking through the foliage we monitor drivers and note how late some of them brake when they come to a blind bend. Most of the cars that pass us fail to brake until they are actually on the bend — with no idea of what is ahead, they are, according to Des, driving dangerously. The two cars that do slow in good time do so, I suspect, because they are curious about what Des and I are up to in the bushes.

* * *

While I am making progress with my driving skills, I am falling behind on my homework (a failing in quite a few of my challenges). But what with my French and my cha-cha practice, I am exhausted at the end of each day. Professor Simons is sympathetic, telling me that the brain uses more energy than any other human organ and since I am taking in — and attempting to learn — so much new information, it isn't surprising that I am so tired. The process of not just writing but *doing* the book has resulted in a dramatic change in my lifestyle; these days, I am often tucked up in bed by 8.30 p.m.

Besides, the driving homework is even more taxing than my French prep.

Not only do I have to implement 'spoken thoughts' every time I drive to Tesco, I am also expected to study the IAM literature and the baffling (not to say boring) Official Highway Code.

'Make that your bedtime reading,' Des suggests.

The only positive thing about this particular home-work is that on the first night I take the Highway Code to bed I don't have my usual trouble dropping off. I think I might have stumbled on a new cure for insomnia! (Sadly, it doesn't last.)

As the weekly lessons go by I gain confidence and, along the way, learn an awful lot more than advanced driving from Des.

'Most people know at some level that driving is one of the biggest killers, particularly in the fifteen to twenty-nine age group. It's another case, like smoking, of what we call cognitive dissonance, when our behaviour conflicts with our beliefs. We know smoking is probably going to kill us, but it doesn't stop us from smoking. You may know that driving is dangerous, but it isn't until something happens to you that you realise how perilous it can be,' he muses during one of our sessions.

Sometimes I completely forget that he is actually, well, Dr Des, until he comes out with some interesting philosophical insight.

'Buddha says from error comes wisdom, meaning we learn from our mistakes, but if you keep repeating those mistakes — which a lot of drivers do every time they get in their car — there is no learning,' he tells me.

Another time he suggests I apply Socratic thinking to overcome a bad habit.

'Socrates' method was to gently challenge knowledge and experience. That's what we do when we ask ourselves "Why do I do what I do?"' he tells me. 'It's at the heart of Cognitive Behavioural Therapy: most problems are habits and what we have to do is first acknowledge those habits and challenge them with Socratic theory. Then we can be mindful of those habits and begin to overcome them. The habit you have got, Jane, is that you do not believe what you are seeing. Your driving is based on what bad thing could happen, which is not a terrible fault, because we want to be able to anticipate things. But if we drive on the basis of what we think might happen rather than what is *actually* happening there is always going to be a delay in our thinking. In other words, we are driving on anxiety, on fear.'

Des's theories are similar to those I have picked up in some of my other challenges and the common message I seem to be getting is to concentrate and remain in the moment.

With Des's help, I am making the kind of progress in my driving that I could never have imagined when I first met him. The grade 2s are now vastly outnumbering the 3s; I feel far more confident and I'm doing my best to implement IPSGA even when I am in a tearing hurry. I have also stopped another bad habit (which I believe I caught off my ex-partner) of being a bit of a bully when another driver is impeding my progress and it isn't possible to overtake. I used to toot my horn and flash my lights, and sometimes, to my shame, would use rude hand gestures. I now know this is counter-productive and cruel (especially when the driver ahead is over eighty and, as they so often seem to be, wearing a hat).

But I face a big obstacle to being 'advanced test ready' because I still haven't confessed to Des my fear of going backwards and, in particular, parallel parking. Somehow during the two months we have been working on my driving I have managed to deflect Des every time he suggests we do a session on 'slow manoeuvring'.

It's time to fess up, and I tell Des an anecdote from my early driving years. Whenever I was driving with my husband in the passenger seat (usually to and from a social event at which he would be drinking) he had a stock phrase that he'd reel off when I parked.

'It's OK, Jane,' he would say as he opened the passenger door. 'I'll catch a cab to the kerb.'

Des, who is something of a feminist, happily married to a woman with a formidable career of her own, comments that the old gender war is still raging on the road.

'Interestingly, I've noticed that most of the women I have taught are lacking in confidence and quite a few of the men that I teach tend to be overconfident. It's as if men can't shake off that sexist old term of abuse "Women Drivers!", when statistically women are the safer drivers,' he says.

Indeed, while there are almost equal numbers of men and women drivers (54 per cent are men), the disparity between the number of motoring offences committed by men and women is startling. The most recent (2018) DVLA figures confirm this, with men taking 7.7 million of the 10.6 million penalty points issued in the last two years. Men are involved in 84 per cent of drink driving incidents and men hold 82 per cent of the penalty points issued for inappropriate mobile phone use.

'There is this misconception, which IAM is keen to highlight, that the faster you go the better the driver you are, which is absolutely not true. There are very good reasons for staying within the speed limits and the exceptional drivers are the ones who can smoothly move through the limit changes and adjust their speed when it is appropriate,' Des informs me.

A crucial thing I learn in my advance driving lessons is to be judicial about speed limits, because quite often roads that have a 60 mph limit, particularly in country areas, can have dangerous bends that can make going at more than 40 mph hazardous.

'Rule 125 in your Highway Code, Jane: "The speed limit is the absolute maximum and does not mean it is safe to drive at that speed irrespective of conditions,"' Des tells me as we drive to a side street for the final showdown on reversing.

One of the reasons — I think — that I have become so scared of reversing my car into a parking bay is that since I moved to the country it is not a procedure I am often pressured to do. There are no parking restrictions on my country road and the fight for parking spaces is nowhere near as intense, even in the centre of my local town. When I was living in central London five years ago, I became very proficient at parking because it was something I did three or four times in the average day.

'I think you have just got out of practice and it's made you doubt yourself,' Des reassures me.

He picks a quiet place for me to have my first try at parallel parking. And miraculously I manage to reverse in line with the cars behind me.

'You did great,' Des says. 'The only thing I would advise is maybe do it a bit slower. Exaggerate how slowly you go, because then if a car or a bicycle unexpectedly comes past, you can just stop the car. Then resume. Don't think you have to do it in sixty seconds or you won't pass. Don't let yourself be governed by drivers who bully you and want you to do something quickly. We shouldn't be rushed or intimidated. You are not on a timer; take as long as you like and if you are not happy with it, do it again.'

It is while Des is directing me to park in a small space ('much smaller than you would ever have to do in the exam') that I have a Eureka moment. Because Des points out something that had never occurred to me before: my car is *straight* when the Mini symbol on the driving wheel is facing towards me. I have finally realised what I am supposed to do when I am told to 'straighten up'. This, pathetic though it might sound, is a game changer in my relationship with parking. On my second attempt I reverse perfectly into the space and Des applauds.

'There you go, absolutely perfect. That's as good as it gets. This idea that you haven't got spatial awareness is nonsense. Parallel parking as you did today is a core part of advanced driving,' Des comments.

When he fills in my course logbook I get even more Grade 2s, and Des tells me I am getting close to being 'advance test ready'.

'Get lots of practice on your slow manoeuvring — you were excellent today — and do as much driving using IPSGA as you can in different conditions and on roads you are not familiar with. Most important of all, know your Highway Code inside out. Then we will have to think about a date for the test,' he says as we part after my eighth lesson.

'Do I have to take the test, Des?' I ask him in a shaky, plaintive voice because while I now know I am not, as I thought, a terrible driver, I still lack confidence in my ability to parallel park to order. Besides I have never been good in test situations.

'Absolutely not Jane,' Des replies. 'If you are uncomfortable with the idea, don't worry. But passing the test and being an official member of IAM is the real aim of what we have been doing.'

In the end we compromise; Des books me a date far enough in the future for me not to be too scared. And, by the time you read this (fingers firmly crossed) I will have a blue chrome and enamel Institute of Advance Motorists badge clamped proudly to the grille of my mini.

4

SWEET (AND SOUR) MUSIC

In which I learn to progress from Baby Shark to Bach . . .

Another of my harrowing long-term memories involves the piano lessons I took — aged ten — with an ancient woman with a lot of facial hair and a very bad temper. With hindsight, I think she was probably about my age now (or maybe younger), but in those days old age started at about forty-one. Besides, she had that negative approach to life (and some of her pupils) that made her seem a hundred and forty-one.

The lessons took place in a hut in her garden on Saturday afternoons and entirely spoilt my weekends. Not just because of her stern methodology (that metronome still strikes in my head when I think about her), but also because I was not the most dextrous child and I struggled with anything more complicated than 'Chopsticks'.

The furthest I got was Grade 1 (which I failed) and the only thing I could play fluently (by heart in the end) was a simplified version of Strauss's 'The Blue Danube' which remains a party piece to this day.

The lessons came to a dramatic end one Saturday when, in the middle of berating me for not having done my homework, my tutor lost consciousness. She slumped forward onto the piano in such a way that I wasn't sure whether she had fainted or died. I sat stunned for the rest of the lesson until one of my friends (who had the lesson after mine) arrived.

The two of us, shamefully, wondered whether we should just make a run for it or get some help. Wicked girls that we were, we exited the hut and went off to join some other friends in the local woods where we had a hideout. We told no one, but later that evening when we finally went back to our respective homes − this was in that innocent age when children were allowed to go out without adult supervision or some sort of digital tracking device − our parents informed us that our teacher had suffered a heart attack. She was, thankfully, recovering well but sadly wouldn't be able to continue with our lessons. This was a double blessing for us because (a) she hadn't died (we had worried about being charged with manslaughter) and (b) we could give up the piano.

* * *

Fast forward to 2019 and another session in Professor Jon Simons' office.

Short of a magic pill (which the Prof thinks is unlikely to happen in his lifetime), it is impossible to prevent the brain slowly degenerating as our bodies age. But by exercising our brain with new challenges that increase our neuroplasticity, we should be able to maintain our cognitive abilities for longer.

'Another of the particularly helpful things you could do is learn a musical instrument,' Professor Simons tells me.

The sound I make at this suggestion is in no way tuneful. I groan and tell him the story of my ill-fated piano lessons.

'Pick another instrument — the violin, the cello, the harp or even the ukulele. You don't even need a teacher — it's possible to teach yourself almost any instrument online nowadays. The one thing I would suggest is that you learn with a friend, because the competition will help motivate you and this will speed up the learning process,' he says.

Back home I google musical instruments and decide that if I failed Grade 1 on the piano I am unlikely to pass it on the violin, the cello, the harp or even the ukulele. I need to find something simpler, the kind of instrument that children learn in percussion lessons — the triangle, the tambourine or the castanets, perhaps? In the end, I settle on the recorder. After all, isn't that the easiest of instruments?

Now all I need is a recorder, an instruction book (both ordered on Amazon for delivery the next day) and a willing friend with a competitive streak. Once again, Belle is the perfect fit.

At first, she is not very receptive. She is very busy/how long will it take/music wasn't her thing, and so on (and on). Eventually, after a series of begging messages on WhatsApp and a reminder that ballroom dancing wasn't exactly my thing, she agrees and we carve out some time in her manic schedule. Belle is one of those superwomen who not only works full-time on her award-winning website, she also runs a home, a husband, and has two of her four grown-up children currently back in the nest. Quite how she manages to maintain the sort of social life that involves cooking lunch for twelve (extended family, assorted friends, me, etc.) most Sundays is beyond me, but it doesn't stop me from forcing her to join in on my musical challenge (or take regular long gossipy walks with our dogs). Batons at the ready!

Lesson 1: Tuesday 3 p.m.

Location: *The cabin at the bottom of my garden*

We each have a descant recorder and a manual entitled *Recorder from the Beginning (Book 1)*. According to the introduction, it is one of the 'most popular schemes used in many parts of the world', 'assumes no previous knowledge of either music or the recorder' and, best of all, 'has been designed for children aged seven upwards'.

'Perfect for us then . . .' mutters Belle.

The book is virtually an idiot's guide with helpful diagrams, colourful illustrations and step-by-step instructions on everything from how to hold your instrument (page 4) to how to make up your own tunes (page 47). But is this, I wonder, what Professor Simons had in mind when he talked of 'an intellectual challenge'?

For a start, the songs that we will be taught to play have names like 'No More Milk' and 'Little Fly' (Strauss, it's not). The only tune we recognise is 'Old MacDonald' (you know, the one who had a farm), and that is way ahead of our current capabilities (page 30) and looks terribly complicated.

I had imagined the recorder to be a glorified whistle — and everyone knows how to whistle, don't they? (As Lauren Bacall famously explained to Bogart in the film *To Have and Have Not* 'you just put your lips together and blow'). But it's not that simple. The first note we learn — B — involves getting our mouths and tongues in the right position to blow gently into our instruments and saying 'tu'. This, we are informed, is called 'tonguing'(*really*).

For some reason the early work engages the left hand more than the right (regardless of whether you are left- or right-handed). This confused me — but not Belle. By the time I had worked out how to hold my recorder and blow at the same time, she had leapt several pages ahead and was attempting to play a tune (albeit in the single note B).

When we finally managed to play something ('Traffic Jam') in unison using our second new note, A, we completely lost it. We laughed so much we almost had a 'TENA Lady' moment (see Chapter 5). This wasn't just because the sound was so terrible, or even because we made so many mistakes. No, it was because Belle — known for her adult sense of humour — suddenly recalled a mnemonic the girls at her convent school learned to help them remember the lines of the scale *AGBDF*. And no, Belle's didn't go All Good Boys Deserve *Favour*.

An hour and a half later when we got to our third note — G — on page 12 ('Gypsy Dance'), we were making such an awful discordant racket that our laughter had been replaced by a headache. Belle stomped off muttering something about how I 'really owed' her for agreeing to this particular venture. Meanwhile I was beginning to question whether — as childish as it was — learning the recorder might be a bigger test of our friendship than dancing the cha-cha-cha.

* * *

Conclusion: It is much, much harder than it looks. Remembering the finger movements for the different notes (OK so we only learned three: B, A and G) requires a great deal of concentration. So I would say it was *absolutely* intellectually challenging, Professor Simons.

Lesson 2: Thursday p.m.

Location: *Belle's home*

Although we didn't realise it during our first lesson, there is a method underlying the order in which we are learning new notes. In starting out with B then A and G, we develop the ability (well, in theory) to play very simple tunes that are known, in recorder circles, as BAG songs. This is an exciting development because some of these tunes we actually recognise — 'Mary Had a Little Lamb', for example. However, recognition is no guarantee of being able to move our fingers fluently from B to A to G (or G to A to B). Undeterred, we abandon BAGs and skip to note E on page 20, which features in a tune called 'Elephants'.

My attempt at introducing this fourth note isn't a success, because now we are expected to bring in our right hands. Progress, at least for me, is very, very slow. The speed at which I learn, compared to Belle (who is *so* much more dextrous than me), becomes something of an elephant in the room.

Hump, wump, dump, chump, Elephants walk with an awful bump should be simple (it *is* simple), but in the time it takes me to even begin to get the hang of the notes for el-eph-ants (A B A), Belle has mastered it and has gone forward two pages to 'Skateboard Ride'. To be fair, this song does actually have a tune ('Elephants' doesn't), and by the time we part it has lodged in our heads in the way that overplayed pop songs sometimes do. Scientific research (honestly) into 'earworms' suggests that the simpler the tune, the likelier it is to become a 'sticky song', i.e. stuck in your brain.

Musicians (OK, I know we are not quite there yet) are particularly prone to PMTs (perpetual music tracks) repeating in their heads, so Belle and I are bracing ourselves for some of the horrors that lie ahead as we progress through our book ('Old Macdonald' and 'There's a Hole in My Bucket', for example).

* * *

Conclusion: We are beginning to understand the torture we put our children through in the early days of their schooling. Belle's son Jacob (twenty-six), who walked in towards the end of Lesson 2, is traumatised by the sight of our recorders (never mind the awful sound). He claims that he still has nightmares from being made to play a recorder solo of 'Silent Night', aged six, in his school Christmas concert.

Lesson 3: Monday 11 a.m.

Location: *The cabin at the bottom of my garden*

Over the weekend, while staying with friends in Hampshire, I feverishly practised my recorder in their shed (the closest I could get to a soundproof space). I discovered another BAG tune in our book 'Hot Cross Buns' that I recognise but we had both missed and, cunningly, learned it off by heart. When I thought I was as close to pitch-perfect as I am ever likely to get, I recorded it on my iPhone ('Hot Cross Buns! Hot Cross Buns! One a penny, two a penny, hot cross buns!'). On Sunday I send the recording (minus the words) to Belle via WhatsApp with the challenge 'Beat that, Belle'.

Five minutes later she messages me back: 'Three Blind Mice, well done maestro'.

Offended though I am that she doesn't recognise the tune I am playing, I comfort myself with the thought that 'Three Blind Mice' is yet another BAG song with exactly the same beginning B! A! G!/B! A! G! (do sing along).

In sending her this recording I have, of course, laid down the gauntlet. Belle not only grabs it, she turns up for our third lesson having discovered something called youcanplayit.com on YouTube. She starts our lesson by playing 'Twinkle, Twinkle, Little, Star' much better than I can play 'Hot Cross Buns'/'Three Blind Mice', even though it includes a new note – F – that isn't in our beginner's book. I am at once both impressed and resentful.

Now the contest begins in earnest. Although we work together today – mastering 'Old MacDonald' from our beginner's book – it's pretty clear that we will get further and faster if we rehearse on our own and then get together once a week to see who is in the lead in this competition.

* * *

Conclusion: Professor Simons' advice on enlisting a friend to learn with may well have speeded up our progress on our recorders, but since we are both secretly (or rather, *obviously*) very competitive, I'm not sure our friendship will survive the savage race to victory. We make the decision that we will not let the recorder get in the way of any other activities we do together, such as our dog walks and our monthly book club evenings. We will only talk about — and play — our recorders together during our once-weekly progress meetings. Oh, and we throw away our beginner's books.

Week 1: Working apart

On my own, in the cabin at the bottom of the garden, I start to learn slightly more adult tunes, thanks to Belle's discovery of youcanplayit.com. I try 'Ten Green Bottles' and while, after an hour of discordant repetition, I am almost there, it is much harder work than I imagined. Harder, I can't help thinking, than learning Mandarin. Because music is a foreign language to me in rather the same way French is (and look how that went). As a child, I failed to master either piano or *Français*, and it's turning out to be an even greater challenge as an older adult. But the thought of Belle racing ahead keeps me focused, so I move on to 'Let It Go' (from *Frozen*). After a long period of practice, it's almost recognisable — to me, if no one else. The dog, in particular, seems to find it very painful.

But I do gain some kudos for the progress I am making with the recorder when my beloved granddaughter Edie comes to stay. Not only is she entranced by the instrument, she is overwhelmed by my ability to play the most irritating earworm of the moment — 'Baby Shark' (which I find on youcanplayit.com). With its ridiculously repetitive and simple melody, it is the easiest piece I have learned since 'Hot Cross Buns'.

'Annie, you are so clever,' Edie tells me, in a way that makes this whole mad music challenge seem almost worthwhile.

* * *

Conclusion: When Belle and I get together for our weekly update we are both, I sense, a bit cagey. I give her a rendition of 'Baby Shark' (but hold back on 'Let It Go'). Belle, meanwhile, says she has hardly any time to practise and all that she can play — rather well, I discover — is 'My Heart Will Go On' (you know the one, from *Titanic*). We applaud each other enthusiastically, but it is obvious that Belle has won this first week hands down (with her dextrous fingers in exactly the right positions).

Weeks 2–4: Working apart

Belle has disappeared off to Corfu for a three-week holiday, so I am confident that I will be able to catch up. Although she will have more time to practise, I doubt she is going to forego the beach, the pool, or the bar for hours and hours of recorder-playing.

It is during Week 2 (though, taking in our first lessons, we are now a month into our practice) that I discover there is much, much more to the recorder than most people think.

Far from being the easy option, the recorder is an incredibly complex instrument with a rich history in classical music. It only acquired its reputation as a simple entry instrument for six-year-olds in schools in the twentieth century when mass-produced plastic descant recorders made it the most economical way to introduce children to music.

Indeed, there is a theory that what puts most children off (rather than on to) playing other instruments is the fact that their early experience of trying to play 'Mary Had a Little Lamb' or 'Hot Cross Buns' on the recorder was too difficult and sounded so terrible. In the hands of those able to master its complexity, the recorder is a beautiful-sounding instrument (*honestly*).

I strike lucky one day by discovering — almost by accident — Sarah Jeffery, who has a YouTube channel called Team Recorder. From the moment I see Sarah (she is young and attractive and wears lipstick and pretty earrings) 'introducing' the instrument she is passionate about (she studied at the Birmingham Conservatoire and plays professionally), I know I have found my virtual tutor.

Sarah has such an enthusiastic, fresh and grown-up approach to teaching that I feel I have finally escaped the nursery (and songs like 'Old MacDonald') and discovered a completely different instrument. Her presentation is infectious and her explanation of finger-positioning (she explains how to stop leakage — which is when the note is way off key because one of your fingers is not in the correct position) and that odd 'tonguing' thing is a revelation. In fifteen minutes online she has taught me to play Debussy's 'Au clair de la lune' (OK it is easy, but it sounds quite good).

Sarah also gives lots of tips that are absent from *Recorder from the Beginning Book 1*. She suggests that the best way to learn is to play with a music stand (I order one on Amazon for £7.99) and she stresses the importance of posture (particularly for the older pupil). She also gives a demonstration of the right way to breathe to make the sound flow properly.

But when I look at some of Sarah's advanced posts, I can see that playing the recorder can take you as far, musically, as those instruments that are generally accepted as having more depth and being harder to learn (all the ones I rejected in favour of my little recorder). Watching Sara's introduction to the twelve pieces of Telemann's 'Fantasias' (written during the eighteenth century; Georg Telemann was part of the Baroque movement) wakes me up to the difficulties I face in mastering the recorder.

I spend some time researching what Sarah describes as the 'vast repertoire' of the recorder. I listen to Vivaldi's 'Recorder Concerto in C major' and Bach's 'Brandenburg Concerto No. 4' (featuring the brilliant Maurice Steger on the recorder). I discover that professional players have around twenty custom-made instruments that cost about £2,000 each (my plastic descant version cost £6.99). Why didn't I know that the recorder was such an important instrument? And how come no one else in the world seems to realise this either? Because the reaction when I tell people that I am 'studying the recorder' is invariably the same — a snort of amused derision.

I am so fascinated by this previously unknown reputation of the recorder that I send an email to Team Recorder (which Sarah started four years ago) asking if I could meet up with her.

Two days later — by which time I have figured out how to assemble my music stand — I get a reply. Sarah is happy to talk to me, but she is based in Amsterdam with her husband Jon (also a musician). So we set up a FaceTime call in which she will listen to me playing and offer some advice on the best ways to improve.

Face-to-FaceTime, Sarah is as engaging and enthusiastic as she is on her videos. I explain about my book and confess that I originally chose the recorder because I didn't think of it as a proper instrument and I imagined it was the easiest option. Now, after struggling through my beginner's book and discovering along the way just how fast and nimble (physically and mentally) you have to be to play something like 'The Flight of the Bumble Bee' (which Sara teaches on another of her videos), I am beginning to think that the violin might have been a simpler choice.

Sarah laughs and says that she gets irritated by the way people tend to dismiss the recorder as a 'toy'. Overcoming that musical stigma was one of the motivations behind Team Recorder. She is desperate to communicate to the lay community (professional musicians recognise that the recorder is as difficult to learn and as valid orchestrally as any other instrument) that it is much more than an easy entry into learning music.

'A lot of people have this idea that the recorder is a bit rubbish. And it can be, if you don't understand the complexity of the instrument. I compare playing it to tightrope walking: your fingers have to be perfectly balanced to achieve the correct sounds. But when it's played properly it is a little like singing, it is the instrument closest to the human voice,' she tells me.

When Sarah posted her first video on YouTube, her intention was to bring the recorder out of the Conservatoire (and out of the nursery) and show people how amazing it can be. She didn't anticipate the reaction to that initial video. Within weeks, Team Recorder exploded and she now has 53.8K subscribers.

I tell her that I have never been very co-ordinated and that I cannot keep up with faster pieces, but she assures me that if I practise, practise, practise (haven't I heard that enough times already in this project?) it will get easier.

'Even at my age?' I say.

'At any age,' she replies.

Indeed, Sarah is particularly taken with the age factor in my challenge. She thinks that my choice of the recorder was — had I but known it — rather wise, as it will make my fingers more flexible, perhaps protecting me against developing arthritis. It will also fine-tune my motor skills and be — as Professor Simons promised — 'brilliant for the brain'. She urges me to continue my research, because there have been a number of scientific studies into the benefits — for older adults — of playing such an instrument.

We have reached the moment when I am to play to Sarah, which is absolutely terrifying. I have spent the last twenty-four hours rehearsing the few pieces I can almost play fluently in my attempt to work out which one I should perform live to such an awesome professional musician. I reject 'Baby Shark' (despite it being my best so far) and rule out 'Hot Cross Buns'. I am tempted to play 'Let It Go' (my second best) but in the end I opt for 'Au clair de la lune' because, after all, it is Debussy, and I have watched Sarah's YouTube tutorial at least ten times.

The first line (GGG AB A GB AAG), which is repeated, goes well but the third, trickier line, (AAAA E EEE AG FF ED) falls down a bit at the end. (I have a similar problem in moving from E to D in 'Old MacDonald'.)

Sarah is very diplomatic and says I am 'not bad for a self-taught beginner', but my biggest problem is that I am using a descant (also known as soprano recorder) and that I really need to invest in a good alto instead. She recommends (she is entirely unsponsored) that I get a Yamaha Ecodear Alto recorder (which, thank heavens, isn't £2,000 but just under £30 on Amazon). She then asks what method book I am using. I confess that I opted for a children's beginner book in the belief this would be easiest. This, it seems, is a mistake, because it tailors the lessons to the level of a child's understanding – and all those infernal nursery rhymes – rather than offering an adult approach to the instrument. Sarah tells me I would be better with an adult method book and suggests *The Sweet Pipes Recorder Book* (a method book 'for adults and older beginners' £17.95 on Amazon).

I ask her how long it will take me to be eligible to take Grade 1, my secret dream being to pass the grade I had failed on the piano when I was ten.

'It takes the average young learner about a year to reach Grade 1,' she sweetly says. 'But I think it will take a beginner of your age much longer – probably around eighteen months, particularly as you are teaching yourself. Then each further grade – up to eight – will take a minimum of a year each.'

'I'm not sure I'll live that long!' I respond.

What I really need is Sarah as my personal tutor, but I don't live in Amsterdam and in any case I probably couldn't afford it.

'I don't think you should worry about exams,' Sarah reassures me. 'You should just keep practising to the point where you are confident enough to enjoy the music you are making.'

I tell her that I already enjoy one particular piece I have learned, but I don't think she would approve.

'It's not exactly Vivaldi or Bach, and its origins are rather complicated, but you probably know it: "Baby Shark".'

Sarah picks up her recorder and plays a perfect Baroque version of the viral song that brings tears to my eyes. We end the call on a promise to keep in contact and a plea from Sarah to 'spread the word' about the real joys and scope of the recorder.

* * *

Later that day, I decide to follow up on Sarah's advice and do a little more research into the other scientifically proven benefits of playing an instrument for life (or at least to Grade 8).

I discover a study from 2012 headed by Professor Nina Kraus, at the Auditory Neuroscience Laboratory at Northwestern University in Illinois.

It is said to be the first study to provide biological evidence that musicians who have played most of their lives suffer less from age-related hearing and memory loss than non-musicians.

Professor Kraus and her team attached electrodes to the heads of a sample group ranging in age from eighteen to sixty-five who had normal hearing. The electrodes measure how long it takes for the brain to process an auditory signal. The normal ageing process slows that timing, making it difficult to process sounds such as a friend's voice in a crowded restaurant.

The older participants, who had made music a part of their life from the age of about nine, could process the signal almost as well as the younger ones, but the non-musicians were much slower. This indicates that playing an instrument is hugely beneficial to retaining memory and hearing.

'As a musician, you get very good at pulling out important information from a complex soundscape,' Professor Kraus reported, 'whether it's a musical performance or listening to someone speaking in a noisy room. The orchestra is playing and you are pulling out the violin line, or the bass line, or some harmony. You are always pulling out meaningful components from sound and that's really not all that different from hearing your friend's voice in a noisy restaurant. That involves hearing, but it's related to how quickly you can process information and how well you remember it,' she said.

* * *

Conclusion: Although I am late to the party (despite having started to learn music when I was ten), I find Professor Kraus's research encouraging. If playing the recorder can help my memory, and particularly my hearing, I am determined to make it a part of the rest of my life.

Week 8: Progress meeting with Belle

Belle has been back from Corfu for three weeks and although we have walked dogs and gossiped together, we have avoided any talk of our progress on the recorder.

I have failed to raise the subject because I feel a cheat, having found Sarah Jeffery and upgraded my recorder and method book (when we first started I had bought Belle's recorder and beginners book, but I had not done the same with my Yamaha Alto instrument).

I am not sure why Belle is ignoring our recorder playing, but then I remember that I had coerced her into the challenge and it occurs to me that maybe she just enjoyed her holiday and forgot about her instrument. In the end, I broach the subject and ask how her recorder practice had gone in Corfu.

'I took it to the beach one day and was playing at what I thought was a discreet distance from the rest of our party — and the strangers sunning themselves.'

'And?' I asked.

'Well, I hadn't picked the thing up for two weeks — this was the last week — and I thought I would start with my best piece . . .'

'"Twinkle, Twinkle, Little Star",' I finish for her.

'No, no, "My Heart Will Go On", remember — from the *Titanic*. Celine Dion, you know?' she replied.

'And how did it go,' I asked, sensing I was going to have to push her on this.

'The first time I played it, I was a bit rusty, a bit terrible. But I had another go, and another go and honestly it was pretty good.' She paused a moment and looked a little warily at me before continuing. 'Anyway, I finish and walk out of my hiding place, and Ed and all our friends, and a lot of other strangers on the beach, were all standing up cheering and applauding — but mostly laughing,' she said.

Apparently, Ed (her husband) had 'made some joke about how it had gone on, and on, and on for so long he thought he might have a heart attack and die if it didn't stop'.

'And you see Jane, I was so mortified, so humiliated that I threw the recorder in the water. It's probably still floating along somewhere in the Ionian Sea which, honestly, is the best place for it. I give up, you win.'

This is a victory to treasure because I have never beaten Belle at anything. But I don't gloat, or boast about my new enthusiasm for my fancy alto instrument with which I have managed to learn 'The Flight of the Bumble Bee'. I just mumble something about how I have to struggle on because of the challenge for my book.

Two months later

Location: *The cabin at the bottom of my garden*

My whole approach to learning the recorder has changed. Inspired by Sarah, I have seriously bonded with my Yamaha and I have discovered that the recorder is rather cool. I hadn't realised that some of the great bands of the 1960s and 1970s featured the recorder (Paul McCartney, for instance, played the recorder on one of my favourite Beatles songs, 'Fool on the Hill' in 1967 and in the same year the late Brian Jones played the recorder on the Rolling Stones number one hit 'Ruby Tuesday').

Then I found out that a number of well-regarded artists today are using the instrument — the American multi-instrument singer songwriter Joanna Newsom plays recorder, Gotye's huge hit 'Somebody That I Used to Know' features the recorder, and the British Indie band alt-J are also fans.

I like to think that I am slowly but surely improving and extending my repertoire. Only today, as I was playing 'Somebody That I Used to Know' (another earworm song) — my twenty-seven-year-old son walked into the cabin and started listening.

'I hate that song, Ma, but that sounded good,' he said (which is praise indeed from him).

Sarah Jeffery may doubt my chances of passing Grade 1 in under eighteen months but — four months in — I am beginning to think I might prove her wrong. In fact I have already started work on the Trinity College London Grade 1 syllabus for 2020. It's daunting, with pieces by Handel, Bach, Grieg and Galilei, but it also includes my absolute all-time favourite, Elgar's 'Land of Hope and Glory'. I now have serious fantasies about playing it in next year's Last Night of the Proms.

5

SEX AND THE SINGLE (OR MARRIED) SIXTY-SOMETHING

In which I delve into things that some people might find offensive . . .

It is a cold, wet Thursday evening in October and Belle and I are on a Great Western train to Paddington. To look at us, you might think that we were a couple of rather dull women (of a certain age) going on an outing. Belle is wearing a sophisticated cropped jacket with tailored trousers and a pair of fashionable brogues, and I am wearing a midi-dress, my new Zara winter coat and my most sensible pair of shoes. No one else on the train could possibly guess that our destination isn't a concert at the Albert Hall or a play in the West End, but an 'erotic emporium for women' in Shoreditch.

For all sorts of reasons (several of them surprisingly scientific) we are on our way to attend a class called Orgasmic! at Sh!, a woman-only sex shop established twenty-seven years ago (men are only allowed in if accompanied by a woman). After a crowded tube journey across London and a ten-minute walk, we arrive at the address and enter, strangely, through a closed coffee shop next door.

If we looked rather ordinary on that Great Western train, we look absolutely extraordinary inside Sh!. The taboo of entering a sex shop may well have been shattered now that there is an Ann Summers retail outlet in every major shopping centre in the country. But while both Belle and I have, at one time or another, glanced at their window displays (which, due to government guidelines set down in 2012, generally feature saucy underwear and fancy-(un)dress outfits), nothing had quite prepared us for the interior of Sh!. Nor, for that matter, was the woman behind the counter − dressed in a matching basque, thong and suspenders − quite prepared for us.

When I told her that we had come for this evening's class (we were, as women of our sort of age tend to be, half an hour early) she smiled, took my money (it was £35 each − obviously I paid for Belle as part of the deal for her accompanying me) and directed us to the area where the class would take place.

There are about twenty-five empty chairs situated around a series of glass coffee tables on which various mysterious objects have been placed. Belle and I sit down in the back row and look around us incredulously. We like to think that we are, well, women of the world, who have, in gynaecological terms, seen it all (we have seven children between us). But we are baffled by some of the merchandise on display.

To our left is an ornate showcase filled with what resemble Venetian glass ornaments but are in fact glass G-spot dildos (several of which glow in the dark). To our right is an artful display of vibrators, strap-on harnesses (don't ask), and various accessories — from zebra-print nipple tassels to vegan edible condoms.

'What do you think those are for?' Belle whispers, pointing to an arrangement of feather dusters in a variety of colours. Closer inspection reveals that they are Tickle Feather Sticks, 'Sensual wands for teasing and stroking'.

Before I expand on the vast and varied stock of Sh! and the details of our lesson with Evie Fehilly, perhaps I should explain the reasons why Belle and I are here in the first place. Sex, you are probably thinking, can't possibly be one of my challenges to future-proof myself for old age? As the following quote from a 1852 edition of Plato's *The Republic* (originally written about 375 BC) reveals, one of the advantages of old age has long been regarded to be *not* having sex:

> . . . I may mention Sophocles the poet, who was once asked in my presence, 'How do you feel about love, Sophocles? Are you still capable of it?' To which he replied, 'Hush! if you please: to my great delight I have escaped from it, and feel as if I had escaped from a frantic and savage master.' I thought then, as I do now, that he spoke wisely. For unquestionably old age brings us profound repose and freedom from this and other passions.

But scientific studies suggest that there are real health benefits to be had from sexual activity in ageing adults. A 2016 study found that older women who had satisfying sex lives had lower blood pressure (a link to a healthier heart). The North American Menopause Society asserts that regular vaginal sexual activity is important for vaginal health as we age. It stimulates blood flow, helps keep pelvic muscles toned and maintains the length and stretchiness of the vagina (who knew?).

Meanwhile, Carol Rinkleib Ellison PhD, a clinical psychologist and sex therapist and the author of *Women's Sexualities: Generations of Women Share intimate Sexual Secrets of Sexual Self-Acceptance,* insists that all sex — partnered or solo — is beneficial for older women. Ellison interviewed 2,632 American women between the ages of twenty-three and ninety and found that 39 per cent of those that masturbate do it to relax. According to Beverly Whipple, co-author of *The Orgasms Answer Guide,* this is because when a woman orgasms the hormone oxytocin is released from nerve cells in the region of the brain called the hypothalamus into the bloodstream. Orgasm relieves tension as the oxytocin stimulates feelings of warmth and relaxation. At an age when lack of sleep is a growing problem, Ellison discovered in another study of 1,866 women that 32 per cent of them used masturbation for a good night's sleep. (The theory behind this is that orgasms release endorphins that can have a sedative effect.)

Perhaps the most convincing, if somewhat bizarre, evidence that post-menopausal women should maintain a sex life (with their partner or by themselves) comes from Rutgers University researchers Barry Komisaruk and Nan Wise. They asked female volunteers to masturbate while they were lying in an MRI machine that measured blood flow to the brain.

When the women 'orgasmed', the blood flow to all parts of the brain increased, allowing nutrients and oxygenation to get there too. They concluded that an orgasm was more stimulating to the human brain than any intellectual challenge. 'Mental exercises increase brain activity but only in relatively localised regions,' Komisaruk said. 'Orgasm activates the whole brain.'

Dr David Weeks, sixty-five, former head of old age psychology at the Royal Edinburgh Hospital, went even further in extolling the advantages of sex for older adults in his 2013 study. Dr Weeks' research, which involved asking a sample group of men and women questions about their sex lives, revealed that those who looked up to seven years younger than their age claimed to have around 50 per cent more sex than the average person in the forty to fifty age group.

'The stereotype of an elderly person is that when they get their pension and bus pass, they stop having sex and that is not true,' Dr Weeks said. 'Sexual satisfaction is a major contributor to quality of life, ranking at least as high as spiritual or religious commitment and other moral factors, so more positive attitudes towards mature sex should be vigorously promoted.'

I should state here that this challenge is not one that was enthusiastically endorsed by Professor Simons. When I emailed him for a comment about the Rutger's research which claims that having orgasms could be better for my cognitive health than taking up a new language or learning an instrument, he was sceptical. He replied that he was not an expert on sex and the brain (any more than any normal person) and couldn't offer anything useful on the subject. I knew what he meant. There is something a little disturbing — not to mention voyeuristic — about research carried out with volunteers happy to 'activate' their brain in an MRI machine while being observed by scientists.

But then sex has never been *my* specialist subject. I am not what you might call an athletic sort of person and I have never been a sexual athlete. I have only had two boyfriends — I married my first aged twenty-one and after I divorced, twenty-five years later, lived with my second for nine years. Like a lot of women of my generation, my sexual education was virtually non-existent. The only intimate anatomical knowledge about my body that I had managed to pick up before I first had sex came from the instruction leaflet in a box of tampons.

But having looked through the seemingly endless scientific studies of the importance of maintaining a sex life into old age, I realised I couldn't leave the subject out of the book. Which brings me back to Sh!, where Belle and I are about to attend a masterclass in masturbation.

At first sight, Evie Fehilly, our teacher (who describes herself as 'artist, performer, idiot, sex educator and clown) looks refreshingly normal. Dressed in matching top, jeans and boots she is curvaceous and smiley and happy to talk to me before the class starts (albeit in double entendres) about how she came to be such a sexpert.

'I trained very much on the job — I am very passionate about my work so I do an awful lot of homework,' she declares with a grin.

When I explain about the premise of my book and my desire to hold on to all my faculties for as long as I can, Evie (in her late twenties) insists there is no age limit on sex or sex education.

'It's a myth that as you become older you become invisible sexually, that sex stops. We know that there are real health benefits from having orgasms and that keeping sex going in a long marriage is really important.'

I tell her I am divorced and that although I still have 'one day my prince will come' fantasies, the reality is that single attractive men of my age are harder to find than a unicorn or a four-leafed clover. I tell her of the horror of going on a 'mature' dating site where the men who 'liked' my profile were either desperately dull, suspiciously young (looking for a sugar mummy?) or had reached that stage of life where they needed a carer rather than a partner.

'Well, my advice to you is to master masturbating in a mirror, because then you will learn exactly what gives you pleasure. And if you ever meet someone again you will be able to show them exactly what to do and where to go,' she says.

By now (and the lesson proper hasn't started), I am beginning to panic.

'Are we supposed to be doing that tonight?' I ask, aware that, in between displays of phalluses (or should that be phalli?) there are an awful lot of mirrors. Maybe it is time, as old journalistic parlance goes, to 'make my excuses and leave'.

'No, don't worry — you don't have to get your bits out! There are legendary classes where you do, but not here,' Evie reassures me.

The chairs are filling up now and Evie's assistant is offering everyone glasses of Prosecco and cupcakes topped with glacé cherries.

'Don't eat or drink *anything*,' Belle whispers in my ear. 'You don't know where it's been . . .'

* * *

Most of the other pupils are in their twenties and thirties and have come with a friend (in some cases a female partner), but there are, reassuringly, a couple of women who could be as old as forty, and a latecomer, elegantly dressed in cashmere, whom Belle calculates to be 'at least fifty-five'.

In rather the way you might do in an AA meeting, Evie asks us all to introduce ourselves, explain why we have come tonight and tell everyone what we like to call our vaginas. Evie starts us off by saying she is very 'fond' of the word c* * * because (and in a way, I agree with her) it's great that feminists are reclaiming the word for themselves.

The first person to stand up is Clare, who says she is here to learn how to have better orgasms. The woman next to her, Frankie, is here to 'help Clare have better orgasms'. They both plump for 'pussy' as their favourite name for their vaginas (a straw poll at the end of the introductions puts pussy as No. 1).

When it's my turn, I mention that I am from a generation that thinks that masturbation is something that men do (a lot) but there is a stigma about women doing something, er, similar. I am here, I say, to be educated about orgasms (I stop short of admitting that I am not sure I have ever had one). Belle says she is here because I didn't want to come on my own, and that she thought 'vagina was a good name for a vagina'.

A young French woman tells us the *vagin* is referred to as '*chatte*', '*foufoune*' or '*zezette*' in France. (I can't wait to impress Arnaud, my French tutor, when I next see him.)

When we are finished with the introductions, Evie moves on to anatomy. First, she shows us a large picture of The Clitoris. Then she passes round a plastic model of a clitoris (telling us to be careful because one strand of it came off last week and it's only loosely glued back on). Belle thinks it looks like a wishbone from a chicken, and I think it looks like mistletoe.

Next up is a large version of the kind of diagram you still get in boxes of tampons, except this one includes the location of the mysterious G-spot. Oh! The G-spot! The existence of this 'secret seat of pleasure' (as it was once described) has been the source of endless scientific argument since 1944, when it was first identified by German researcher Dr Ernst Grafenburg. In 2003 a University of Sheffield study declared that there was no evidence to support its existence and in 2013, after dissecting the vaginal wall of an eighty-three-year-old cadaver (*ugh*), scientists at the Institute of Gynaecology in St Petersburg Florida 'confirmed' that the G-spot *did* exist (although I can't help but wonder if the poor woman had found it for herself before she died).

Evie is not only certain it exists, she can pinpoint her own in, she tells us, a matter of seconds. (I once wrote a piece for a national newspaper, to my then husband's horror, in which I said that apart from the Holy Grail and my car keys, nothing has been more rigorously pursued than the G-spot, and if it ever did turn up it would probably be in the fruit-bowl or behind the fridge). But I digress, back to class.

To help us identify our G-spots, Evie introduces us to a glove puppet called Ruby Vulva. Ruby is made of different fabrics to represent different anatomical areas of a woman's bits. Ruby's, er, lips are made of shiny scarlet satin, for example, and her G-spot is made of thick corduroy. Evie passes Ruby round the class so that we can all delve inside her to identify that textured material

103

source of pleasure. It is at this point that Belle whispers to me, 'I warn you, it's going to take me a long time to get over this.'

Then Evie passes us each a photograph of one section of Jamie McCartney's *Great Wall of Vagina* — a vast art installation made up of plaster casts he took of over four hundred vulvas.

'Do you recognise yourself in any of these?' Evie asks us. There is an outburst of exclamations as various women point to one or other plaster cast, but Belle and I stay silent.

Moving on (the lecture was nearly two hours), Evie gives us tips on what she calls 'solo play'.

'Plan to see it as a lovely long evening of pleasure just for yourself. Take time, remember the brain is the biggest erogenous zone in the body, so stimulate it, use porn, audio erotica — whatever you like. Make yourself a masturbation playlist — classical music works really well for me because it often builds slowly to a fantastic crescendo.'

I was hoping that after Evie had particularly recommended Tchaikovsky's *1812 Overture* we would be free to leave, but no. Evie then introduces us to various sex toys (all available with a 20 per cent discount tonight). There are hundreds of them, in all shapes, sizes and colours, offering different levels of battery- and Bluetooth-operated *thrusts* and *vibrations*. On quiet days in the shop, Evie's assistant tells us, they sometimes have a Dildo Derby, racing them across the floor.

Evie holds up something that looks like a large microphone and tells us it is a version of the Magic Wand that Hitachi innocently launched in the 1960s as a muscle massager.

'The story goes that when they discovered people were using it to masturbate, they stopped making it. But you can still buy magic wands — and this one speaks to my soul,' Evie swoons.

Then there is a selection of the aforementioned glass dildos, various versions of 'The Pebble', silver, gold and bronze handbag-sized 'Bullets' and a . . . well, an instrument that Evie says is particularly 'fast' and brilliant.

'The only trouble with this,' she says, looking directly at me, 'is that it has strong magnets within it and you can't use it if you have a pacemaker.'

The noise of the different gadgets whirring and throbbing is beginning to give me a headache and, as we are about to move on to those strap-ons, I stand up and say that we have to leave to catch our train. We don't even buy anything. I had intended to get something to complete my solo sex challenge, but the only thing I liked the look of — the discreet We-Vibe Wish Pebble Vibrator (with Smartphone control and ten modes) — was £119.

An hour later, when we are safely seated in our comfort zone (a near-empty Great Western train), Belle and I cry with laughter as we replay certain moments of our evening. Belle can't wait to share the highlights of our orgasmic lesson with her husband, but I go home feeling not the slightest desire for solo play, particularly in front of a mirror . . .

* * *

Having failed in my attempt to find my G-spot and have multiple orgasms (I am *still* not sure what an orgasm is), I do some additional research into sex and the older woman. It seems the key word for women who, like me, are out of practice (blush), or suffer from post-menopausal vaginal dryness, is *lubrication.*

'Lubricant is an awful word, isn't it? It doesn't have very positive connotations,' says Sarah Brooks, one of the two founders of the Yes Company, which produces certi-fied organic, natural vaginal moisturisers, lubricants and washes. 'We tried to think up another word for it like *Luberation* that would be more positive, but we gave up.'

Sarah, a chemist, and her friend Susi Lennox, an English graduate, came up with the idea for the Yes Company in 2003, prompted by their experience working in different divisions of Pfizer when Viagra was launched in 1998.

'We became aware of a social side effect that Viagra was having on older women whose husbands were taking the drug and becoming sexually active for the first time in years,' Sarah says.

The letters page of the *New York Times*, she tells me, was overrun after the launch of the little blue pill by women writing in, saying things like, 'my husband and

I haven't made love for twenty years and suddenly he wants sex every night', or 'When my husband started to take Viagra he became very sexually demanding and I couldn't cope. Now he's run off with a twenty-year-old.'

They realised that the sexual boost Viagra gave to the male libido was having an adverse effect on their female partners. It's estimated that 50−80 per cent of menopausal women experience vaginal dryness due to declining oestrogen levels, but the only products available at that time were synthetically formulated − often containing ingredients such as parable preservative and propylene glycol, which are known to have harmful effects on the body and particularly on highly sensitive intimate tissues.

Sarah and Susi could see that there was a growing gap in the market for a range of intimacy products that were gentle, free of chemicals that were known to be skin irritants, and, most importantly, effective. It took them three and a half years to research and develop their products, and to fund the business start-up they both sold their homes. Their mission, they say, was to 'change the world from the inside'.

Since their launch in 2006, the Yes range has become so successful that it is now sold in ninety-three countries, with UK stockists including Sainsbury's and Superdrug (you can order them on Ocado too). Two of their products are also available on prescription on the NHS for women suffering from vaginal atrophy (the thinning, drying and inflammation of the vaginal walls) that is most common in menopausal women and can make sex painful.

Sara believes that part of their success is down to the way they have designed their packaging, which is discreet, subtle and 'respects the sensitivity of the people who buy it. We wanted to get rid of any feeling of embarrassment that older women might have experienced in the past when they put one of the old-style intimate products in their shopping trolley'.

Funny, charming and informative, Sara tells me more about female anatomy than Evie the sex educator managed in two hours. She quotes the conceptual artist Sophia Wallace, who in her pioneering Cliteracy TED Talk in 2015, commented, 'How is it possible that we landed on the moon and walked around on it twenty-nine years before discovering the anatomy of the clitoris?'

It wasn't until 1989 that the Australian Urologist Helen O'Connell revealed the true size and scope of the clitoris. By creating an internal map she discovered its massive size and huge amount of nerve endings (8,000 compared to the 3,000 of the male penis). The clitoris in its entirety is roughly the size of the penis and it also contains erectile tissue.

Sarah plays down the role she and Susi have played in helping women suffering from vaginal atrophy, not to mention all those Viagra widows who have been able to enjoy sex again. 'It's fantastic when we get emails and calls from happy customers. We call them "Yestimonials", and we got one recently from a couple who were both a hundred years old, thanking us for helping them to have sex again. I didn't ask them for the details . . .'

* * *

The most positive result of this chapter, and what you might call my own Yestimonial, wasn't discovering that 'penis envy' is a thing of the past now that we know we have one too (just on the inside rather than the outside). Nor was it finding out that sex is good for your health whatever your age. What really helped me was undergoing a twelve-week course to retrain my pelvic floor muscles. Not, you understand, on the off-chance that one day my prince *will* come (I've gone off that idea after the worrying talk about 'love balls', Kegel exercises and marbles at Sh!) but to prevent me from suffering bladder leaks — a problem that one in three women experience from time to time as they age. I don't want to turn into a TENA Lady before my time.

It wasn't as if I had a serious problem, but sometimes, mostly on riotous wine-fuelled nights out with girlfriends, I would find myself so overcome by laughter that I was suddenly overwhelmed by an unbearable urge to, well, *wee*.

On one such night a girlfriend and I were struck with the same affliction at the same time and we had a race, doubled over in an attempt to control our bladders, to the one loo at the local Pizza Express. To my shame, I pushed ahead of her, slammed the door in her face, and just about made it. She didn't.

There have been other such moments in other situations. At the beginning of my gym challenge (see Chapter 10) I ran into trouble, particularly during track training, when a sudden vigorous movement (star jumps) caused me anxiety. Then again, from time to time out on a dog walk a violent sneeze could have a worrying effect on my bladder control.

So although it wasn't an everyday occurrence of what I believe they call 'clinical incontinence', it was embarrassing enough for me to sometimes buy a box of one of the various brands of 'discreet' pads that get bigger the greater the problem might be (thankfully I only ever needed the slimmest, for 'light leakage').

With the changing demographic — all those ageing baby boomers needing protective bloomers — the market for such products is predicted to explode over the next few years. There are already six million male and female adults in the UK suffering from serious incontinence problems, and one in four are women over the age of thirty-five.

TENA, one of the brand leaders, recently launched a range of disposable Silhouette pants (called Noir) with 'triple protection', designed and advertised specifically to make them look fashionable (and sexy). In one, a mum in her thirties (pregnancy and childbirth are a cause of incontinence in younger women) is wearing the black Silhouette pants with a push-up black bra while saying, 'A little bit of wee is not going to stop me being me.'

In another, an older — pretty but probably post-menopausal woman — says 'one of the good things about getting older is knowing what you want'. She is then shown out shopping with her adult daughter, who tries to persuade her to buy a knee-length pencil skirt. 'I don't think so,' the mother says at the end of the ad as she walks down the stairs, dressed to go out in a short skirt and high heels. 'Not because of my incontinence — I just prefer minis.'

Looking way back to the foggy days after the birth of my first child, I vaguely remember being given instructions about exercising my pelvic floor muscles. But exercising anything with a newborn (my brain in particular) was impossible. Two more babies and three decades later, it seemed like a good idea to undergo one of the many pelvic muscle retraining systems on the market to ensure that my 'light' leakage didn't develop into an uncontrollable torrent.

Having researched various 'electronic pelvic exercisers', I chose Pelviva, not just because it claimed to have developed a 'life-changing technological breakthrough' for weak bladders, but because it was cheaper than the other — scary-looking — products on the market (which can cost anything between £118 and £250 — my Pelviva starter pack cost £42).

Each of the individual exercisers — which resemble a large white plastic tampon, complete with an exit string — comes with a sachet of lubricant. You insert them as you would a tampon, leaving them in for half an hour (the point at which the 'reactive pulse technology' stops working) before disposing of them. When I first used one, I found the effect of the pulse mildly alarming (but not painful and certainly not *arousing*). Although it is perfectly possible to walk around and carry on as normal when you are using one, I chose to take half an hour out (I work from home) to go to bed with a book.

The reactive pulse (that comes from a microprocessor within each retrainer) works on both types of muscles in the pelvic floor: the power muscles that help prevent leaks when you cough, sneeze or star jump, and the endurance muscles that help you hold on when you urgently need the loo.

Every other day for twelve weeks I used the pelvic muscle retrainer, and the effect was noticeable within a fortnight. I discovered that I no longer needed discreet 'light leakage' pads when star-jumping in the gym. Interestingly, although this could just be a placebo effect, I have also stopped getting up to go to the loo at night.

Three months on, having added some simple daily exercises to maintain my muscle control, I feel confident that I will sail through to my seventies and beyond without the need to buy a pack of sexy Noir Silhouette pants (with their triple action control). I am, I like to think, facing the future feeling absolutely *watertight.*

6

AQUA-FLEX

In which I learn to throw in the towel (and get back in the water) . . .

As, er, watertight as I now am, I don't swim if I can possibly help it. I *can* swim, quite well, as long as I don't get my hair wet. But swimming was never going to be an exercise of choice in my bid to future-proof my ageing body. In the last couple of years I have reluctantly swum a length or two of breaststroke on about four occasions, pressurised by my mocking adult children on holidays.

But when I began to plan this book it became obvious that swimming was probably the best low-impact exercise I could do. When the UK Chief Medical Officer published a revised MVPA (Moderate-intensity and Vigorous-intensity Physical Activity) list for older adults in September 2019, it featured prominently.

Despite that, the idea of joining a swimming club or enrolling in an aqua aerobics class filled me with horror. Not, you understand, because I am scared of water (as many mature adults probably are) but because, shamefully, I am scared of wearing a swimming costume in a public place.

As a result of this pathetic inhibition I have developed a curious way of covering myself up whenever I cannot avoid entering a swimming pool.

This involves me emerging from the changing room wrapped in a large towel that I will leave as close to the top of the pool steps as I can. The towel functions as a kind of comfort blanket, so that no one will see me *full length* in my one-piece before I am submerged. Then I have to plan my exit from the pool, waiting until I think no one is looking and then making a grab for my comfort towel as soon as I reach the top step before I run as fast as I can back to the changing rooms.

This absurd behaviour probably developed when I was a teenager, years before the term 'fat shaming' had become a thing. It's an age at which so many women (look back on your own youthful pictures) begin to *fat shame* themselves into a kind of collective body dysmorphia. If your body didn't line up with that of the supermodels of your day, you decided you were fat. How could I possibly imagine my eighteen-year-old body was — well, normal — when it didn't measure up (in width or height) to that of, say, Christie Brinkley (who is set to look as ridiculously perfect in her seventies as she did back in the seventies)?

As a thirty-something, contented, size-14 mum, I still longed to look like Kate Moss (whose words 'nothing tastes as good as skinny feels' still leave a sour taste in my mouth). Normal, in the last few decades, has become the new fat.

Surely, you might think, a sixty-something woman (a granny, for goodness' sake) must have left all that self-obsessive nonsense behind her? Yet only last summer — after my elder daughter had invited me to join her and friends on a villa holiday in France — I found myself fretting for weeks beforehand about being — as the saying goes — *beach body ready*. And although I knew that by now I should be mature enough not to care about all that ridiculous nonsense about cellulite, six-pack abs and taut tummies, I have to admit that it still bothered me. Why, before I bought a (rather too daring for my liking) yellow Secret Slimming Marks and Spencer costume (the only one left in my size) I had seriously considered trying to get hold of a full-body burkini.

It was on that holiday that my daughter introduced me to both the concept of Body Positivity and the Patriarchy (OK, so I am a bit late getting to both), and prompted me to question my madness.

She waited until one afternoon, when the two of us were alone in the pool, to challenge me.

'Mum,' she mused from a flamingo water float on which she was lying looking magnificent in a red-and-white striped bikini, 'why do you do that thing with your towel?'

'What thing?' I snapped.

'That thing of dropping the towel a second before you get into the pool and picking it up again the second you get out?' she continued. 'It's almost as if you think your body is in some way disgusting, when in fact it's

115

miraculous. You shouldn't care whether other people think you look amazing, because your body is amazing — it keeps you alive every day. And it gave birth to me.'

I should perhaps mention that my daughter Bryony is something of a legend for her work in mental health and the way she has furthered the cause of Body Positivity. She has single-handedly turned the idea of the picture-perfect Instagram post on its head by regularly putting up unfiltered pictures of herself pouting in her size 18 underwear or her brand-new low-cut bikini. She often has a pop at my generation of mothers who, from her view as a child, constantly fretted about how they looked and how much they weighed. But, as we floated round that infernal pool, I became aware that she was going to question me about my other silly swimming foible.

'And why on earth are you so obsessed about getting your hair wet?' she declared. 'Honestly, in my whole life I have never seen your natural hair. You are always so perfectly coiffed with blow-dried hair that you go to ridiculous lengths NOT to get wet. What are you afraid of?'

'Looking like a blonde Brian May,' I reply.

'Let's see it then — I dare you!' she continues, in such a commanding way that — for the first time in at least forty years — I swim half a length underwater.

When I emerge, Bryony is standing on the side of the pool taking pictures of me on her phone. Pictures that are then posted to to our family WhatsApp with the caption: 'Shock, horror, Mum gets her hair wet!'

Strangely, I rather like the way I look in them, which only encourages Bryony to go on torturing me.

'You are in thrall to the Patriarchy, Mum. Let your hair be naturally beautiful and for f*ck's sake throw in the bloody towel,' she concluded on that fateful summer day.

Whether or not it is the Patriarchy that has made me so negatively body conscious is debatable (I am as nervous in front of other women as I am in front of men), but my idea of hell during the time of my life when I probably *was* beach body ready (had I but known it) was wearing a bikini on a beach. And for the following four decades, I have allowed the ridiculous notion of being judged for how I looked in a swimming costume prevent me from doing something that I had loved when I was a child. What was I thinking? Who did I imagine was watching me? And why had I spent my entire adult life straightening my thick, naturally curly hair?

And, oh, how I regretted all those lost summer holidays when my children were growing up and I had mostly been a poolside observer, rather than a participant, in their water fun and games.

When I returned from that holiday I began to think about adding swimming to the list of things I could do to strengthen my body. My attempt to become a bona fide gym bunny with Ash, my brilliant but brutal personal trainer (see chapter 10) was already well under way, along with FitStep dancing classes with Belle, but progress was slow. In truth, I found both of these to be harder work (physically) than I was comfortable with.

Those misgivings were outweighed by the undeniable health benefits of swimming. Research has proven that it can make your heart stronger by boosting cardiovascular strength and lowering your blood pressure. Along the way, regular swimming (which puts every muscle group in the body to work) can improve circulation and help reduce the risk of lung disease. Moreover, because it's not weight bearing, it is ideal for older people with arthritis and general joint pain or discomfort.

There is also reason to believe that senior swimming can improve bone mineral density (BMD) which helps fight osteoporosis, a condition that causes one in three women and one in five men to suffer bone fractures. Other benefits include increased flexibility in your hips, legs, arms and neck; and because it is an exercise that improves your posture, it can be helpful for people who suffer from back pain. On top of that, it's a great way to reduce your stress levels, improve your mood and increase your brain function. When pursued as a social activity, swimming can lessen feelings of isolation and loneliness that can lead to depression in older people. Adding it all up, I decide that this is a challenge I dare not avoid any longer.

There was, however, one lingering scruple, aside from my reluctance to wear a swimming costume in public. I have always been squeamish about leisure centre pools. You know what I mean: shower drains clogged with human hair, plasters and chewing gum (several years ago the closest public pool to me had its failings exposed — in disgusting, graphic photographs — in our local paper).

Despite my reservations, I found a leisure centre within a twenty-mile radius of my home that was rated 'clean and friendly', and bravely turned up one Monday morning for a Water Workout (another term for Aqua Aerobics) with a teacher called Cindie. There were about twenty-five women of varying ages, shapes and sizes in the pool; a few young mums, a clutch of pre-menopausal women and some post-menopausal women like me. So, even though I still couldn't let go of my comfort towel, I was in what you might call good company. Apart, that is, from our nineteen-year-old instructor, whose body did match up to the supermodel of her day. Cindie was a fake-tanned clone of Kylie Jenner (at twenty-two the youngest Kardashian *and* the youngest 'self-made' US dollar billionaire).

It wasn't her looks that upset me (honestly), but her bored and slightly aggressive approach to the class. Oh, and the garage music she played, over which it was all but impossible to hear her shouting out instructions and repeatedly screaming 'Faster!' and 'Harder!'

Later that day at one of my gym sessions with Ash, I told him about my miserable experience. He laughingly recalled the time he worked in a spa where they had to measure the water levels in the swimming pool every two hours.

'We noticed a significant jump in combined chlorine levels after an aqua aerobics class. That tells you the sanitising effect of the chlorine has been substantially reduced by the number of human bodily excretions released into the pool. Many people don't shower before they swim and then of course they are sweating and, yes, I am afraid — particularly after classes of older people — there would be a lot of pee in the pool.'

Ash, who is at the top of his profession and somewhat disparaging about the physical benefits of swimming, insists that it can only be 'good exercise' if I do it fast enough and long enough. Even then, he says, it's not going to help with building my bone density in the way that my strength-training sessions with him will.

'You need to swim about seventy-five lengths as fast as you can to get the kind of benefit that you would get from cross-training in the gym,' he tells me.

This is probably an exaggeration, but it is true that swimming at an easy pace for one hour burns fewer calories than exercises such as running and cycling. Nor does the endurance you build up in swimming raise your endurance in other activities in the way that some other exercise forms do.

The following week I attempt to take Ash's advice on swimming (that it is only good exercise if it is fast and involves at least a non-stop hour in the pool) and pay £20 for an entry pass to one of the fashionable, newly renovated lidos that are opening up all over the country. This particular establishment doesn't just offer all-year-round swimming and glamorous spa treatments, it also boasts a beautiful restaurant where you can eat 'exquisite' tapas in a glass-walled area overlooking the pool.

Thankfully, I had brought my own towel (bath-sheet size) so I didn't have to hire one of their smaller £3 ones. Because, let me tell you, getting into that pool to swim lengths in front of around a hundred cool young diners was really, really scary. The idea of them eating their Wood-Roasted Scallop starters (£12.50), their Seared Sirloin of Beef Caponata Basil and Aged Parmesan main courses (£23) while they watched me attempting (and of course failing) to swim seventy-five lengths, brought my lido experience to a premature end. I managed exactly four lengths before grabbing my towel and leaving.

* * *

I would probably have given up on swimming my way to a healthier, stronger body if I hadn't — almost by chance — discovered the incredible Dee Keane. Dee, who is sixty-two, has designed a swimming system specifically for adults over fifty-five. She has a long history with the sport, having spent fifteen years teaching the Shaw Method. Created in the 1980s by Steven Shaw, who applied the proven principles of the Alexander Technique (created to retrain habitual patterns of movement and posture) to swimming. Partly inspired by the experience of caring for her mother — who died five years ago in her mid-eighties — Dee began to think of ways in which gentle exercise in water could help people retain their mobility and strength as they age.

'Aqua-flex is a mixture of stretches and warm-ups, the sort of thing you would do with any physical activity. It involves some cardiovascular work, a little yoga breathing, some pelvic-floor movements and muscle-strengthening exercises that are specifically helpful to anyone fifty-five and over. But what we work on the most is building up our strength in our non-dominant sides, which is hugely important as we age,' she tells me.

Dee explains that, for the majority of the population, our right side thinks it should run the world and our left side likes this because it thinks it doesn't have to do anything. This is fine when we are young and fit, but dangerous when we reach an age when we don't just fall over — we *have a fall*.

According to Age UK, falls are the most frequent and serious type of accident in people aged sixty-five and over. In people over seventy-five, falls are the main cause of disability, and the leading cause of death from injury.

It has long been established that any kind of physical activity can lower the risk of a fall, but research conducted by the University of Western Sydney in 2014 suggests that swimming is the only exercise that can genuinely lower the risk in the over-sixties. Based on a sample of 1,700 men aged seventy assessed over a four-year period, researchers concluded that swimmers were 33 per cent less likely to suffer a fall. They also performed better in a test of 'postural sway', which measures how much your body moves while standing still for thirty seconds.

If you do fall, Dee points out, it will be your dominant arm or leg that you will break or injure, and your left side will have to 'step up to the mark'. But it won't be able to unless you have worked on it. And building up your non-dominant side doesn't only help after a fall, it improves your overall strength and balance, making you less likely to fall over in the first place.

By now I am ready to sign over my life — and my left non-dominant side — to Dee. But first I tell her about my lifelong loathing of being seen in a swimming costume.

'For a lot of people a swimming pool is not a comfort zone. It is uncomfortable, intimidating, embarrassing,' she assures me, before telling me about an Aqua-flex class that she runs at a gated community for older people in Oxford. 'You will be inspired by these amazing women to overcome any inhibition you have,' she continues. 'A lot of these women have mobility problems and were very unsure at first, but what they learned very quickly is that they feel better in the water because movement is so much easier. They keep coming because they can do things with their bodies in water that they could not do on dry land,' Dee says.

* * *

Which is why, the following Wednesday, I find myself in the Pegasus Grange swimming pool with nine other women, waiting for my first Aqua-flex class to start. The heating is turned up in the poolside area to tropical

123

levels, and the water is, at least for me, rather too close to bath temperature. But looking out through the big windows I realise how cold and wet it is today and I give an involuntary shiver.

Lined up alongside me — clutching the rail on one side of the pool as we warm up — are Val, ninety-seven; Toni, eighty-one; Little Pat, eighty-seven; and Big Pat, seventy-four. On the other side, closer to Dee, are five other swimmers, all ready to go.

Being allowed to attend the class is something of an honour. For a start, I had to have the approval of all nine women (who own flats in Pegasus Grange, which lies in the heart of the city of Oxford). Swimmers like Margot, a smiling ninety-two-year-old with limited sight, and Pam, eighty-seven, who informs Dee that she won't be here next week as she is 'off on a Caribbean cruise'.

'You're not cruising *again*, Pam,' comments Dee, prompting a chorus of laughter from the rest of the class.

Allowing a sixty-something whippersnapper like me to join them in the pool is really generous because I am probably the only one here who hasn't got a medical problem or two. They have no idea, Dee assures me, about my ridiculous psychological swimming disorder and my 'comfort towel', which, for the first time ever I have left in the changing room.

The only thing that is making me uncomfortable so far is the realisation I am the only one who is not wearing a modest plain black regulation swimsuit (yes,

I am back in my yellow Secret Slimming Marks and Spencer costume).

'Right, ladies,' says Dee, because, she tells me later, they belong to a generation that still regards calling them 'women' as rather rude. 'Let's start with some walking on the spot, gradually working up to some jogging.'

I had assumed that I would find this particular class of Dee's a breeze, but at times I find it difficult to keep up.

'Now, ladies, let's do some big stretches. Stand up on your toes — as if you are wearing your highest stilettos — and then lower yourself back on the ball of your foot,' she instructs, as Big Pat pulls herself up a foot higher than I can.

We roll our shoulders one way, then the other, and we pull them up to our ears and down again. We walk backwards across the pool (good for our spatial senses). We fast jog, we walk our legs up the wall, we do a lot of non-dominant side work and we build up our grip by squeezing some hand-and-wrist gel resistance balls.

'Come on, ladies,' Dee commands. 'Squeeze those balls really tight, because if we lose our grip we are in big trouble. I mean, how are we going to be able to open a bottle of wine? Let's get our priorities right.'

What is impressive about Aqua-flex is that it involves working on every muscle in your body, even the ones you didn't realise *were* muscles.

'Right, now we're going to do our eyeball exercises that help us preserve our sight. Those tiny, tiny muscles in our eyes that can just pack up as we get older. Revolve your eyeballs all the way round — and now the other way. Repeat . . .'

The class joke, though, is the very last muscle we need to get moving.

'Come on now, altogether let's work on those *tongues*,' Dee says, and with almost precision timing the class poke their tongues in and out in a way that, oddly, reminds me of a warped kind of synchronised swimming.

It isn't until we get out of the pool that I realise Margot cannot move at all without her walker (as Zimmer frames are now known), and that, without water to support her, Val needs a rather chic walking stick to get around.

While we wait for the showers (there are only two), eighty-one-year-old Toni, a tall elegant woman with a youthful gamine haircut, chats to me about how Aqua-flex has boosted her confidence and her strength.

'I was one of those people who never had anything wrong with me, never went to the doctors, then one day — just over two years ago now — I woke up and I couldn't move my hands, I couldn't grip anything. It was terrifying. In the end I had a neck operation — the spinal column was being squashed.'

Toni is a retired art teacher and the thought that she might not be able to use the hands that had played a vital part in her much-loved professional life was devastating.

'I was such a healthy person that it came as a terrible shock,' she tells me. 'And of course it affected my confidence. I was so weak on one side that I was terrified of falling, which is why I started these classes. I wasn't a swimmer and I didn't realise how wonderful it was to be in water, and how it could help me be stronger and more flexible. And such fun,' she adds.

As we talk, Little Pat, who is the last to come out of the pool, exclaims as she stands holding on to the rail at the top of steps, 'Oh, I feel so *heavy* now.'

It isn't until she says this that I realise how true it is. I hadn't ever connected that feeling you get when you reach for the bars to pull yourself out of the water with the fact that one of the greatest pleasures of swimming is the sensation of weightlessness. It is, I suppose, the closest we can get on earth to floating in Space.

Dee tells me that often the older women in Aqua-flex classes are amazed by how good they feel once they are able to relax in the water.

'Once they learn that water will hold you, that you don't have to do anything other than float, it is such a liberation. For the older classes it feels more comfortable than lying in bed. The water embracing you and holding you is a glorious feeling, once you switch off your muscles and relax. For many people in their eighties, the idea that they can stand on one leg or bring their knees up to their chests is unimaginable. From our fifties and sixties we all start to slump, so holding yourself up straight can be difficult. But the water will support you, and you can't slump because you're trying not to drown!'

As I drive home after my first class (I am now a regular and well bonded with the other Pegasus Grange girls) I feel brilliant. I was not aware that I too had begun to slump and I am conscious that — on dry land (as Dee always says) — I need to hold up my shoulders and walk tall. The biggest benefit, though, is that the classes have made me fall in love with swimming the way I did when I was a child.

I had forgotten how wonderfully light and agile you feel in the water and how your body can do things you can't do anywhere else (not even the bath). It's almost as if I have super-powers in water, as if I could be (as I used to make-believe when I was five years old) a mermaid. Especially now, when I am quite happy putting my head underwater and having mermaid — rather than Brian May — hair.

Experiencing this uplifting sensation alongside a group of women twenty and thirty years older than I am somehow adds to this liberating feeling. Watching Val doing star jumps with the ease of a young woman — despite being very frail, with a hearing aid and two hip replacements — is inspiring. It is also humbling; my Aqua-flex classes haven't just been physically exhilarating (and, by the way, hilarious), they have been brilliant for my mental health and confidence. And, yes, since joining Dee's class I have abandoned that mad comfort towel routine. As my daughter said, my body is amazing and it doesn't matter what anyone else might think about it. What's more, with a once-a-week Aqua-flex class my body will, fingers crossed, keep me alive every day until I am ninety-seven like Val.

It is Dee's dream to one day roll out Aqua-flex classes across the country and to put pressure on the government to ensure that every purpose-built facility for older people has a swimming pool.

'I am really passionate about this. Sadly, not enough old people have access to a swimming pool, and swimming is one of the very few ways you can maintain your mobility and agility as you age. Not to mention the fact that it is, in an age when loneliness is such a blight on the lives of older people, a fantastic form of social contact,' she says.

I realise that my new swimming regime is not going to build my strength in the way that some of my other physical challenges — weightlifting and boxing with Ash and ballroom dancing with Ian Waite — are doing, but it is building up my non-dominant side (I can now open a bottle of wine with my left hand). And I have finally discovered that, in water, everyone is ageless and weightless.

7

MEDITATION AND MINDFULNESS

*In which I overcome my scepticism about all things
Zen and WOKE myself up . . .*

There is so much noise in my head that I can't sleep.
Most nights I am still struggling to 'drop off' at 2 a.m.,
having done everything I can think of to stop the whirring, crashing and pinging that is going on in my brain as
it attempts to process what it tried to learn the previous
day. And when I do finally slip into unconsciousness, I
have the strangest dreams that are haunted by French
verbs, dance moves, sheet music and the 307 rules in
the Highway Code.

By 10 a.m. each morning, high on caffeine, I am
finding it difficult to concentrate and beginning to doubt
my ability to achieve any of the goals I have set myself.
I need, I realise, something that will help me relax, calm
the madness in my head and — most importantly —
allow me to sleep.

It is Belle who, as it were, wakes me up to the need
to find some respite for my over-stimulated cerebrum.

'This brain and body work you are doing is all very well,' she says to me one day when we are out walking our dogs 'But what are you doing for your mental well-being? What are you doing to relax?'

I tell her about the box sets of French crime dramas I am watching in the evenings (in the hope that reading the subtitles and listening to the dialogue will help me absorb the language) and the various brain-games I do in my daytime downtime. She gives me a withering look and informs me that what I need – and what she is about to embark on – is a course in mindfulness and meditation. This, she insists, will do as much to help me *not* get old as any of my other challenges.

'It's a series of talks over five weeks by this brilliant man who is a Zen Buddhist teacher. It will completely change your life. I will sign you up and send you over the list of the health benefits of meditation. You won't believe it,' she tells me.

I am pretty sure that, she's right: I won't believe it. When she sends the documents over in an email later that day, my first thought is 'this *is* unbelievable'.

There is something for everyone on this list of the seventy-nine physical and mental benefits of meditation. Not only can it cure temporary insomnia (my current complaint) it can also reduce road rage, end migraines, lower cholesterol levels and blood pressure, build strength, make you sweat less (?), make you more fertile (too late for me). But these are the benefits – if true – that pique my interest:

No. 20: Decreases the ageing process. (What's not to like? Although it doesn't say how.)

No. 21: Higher levels of DHEAS (Dehydroepiandrosterone. (This, I discover, is a hormone that produces other hormones such as testosterone in men and oestrogen in women. Our DHEAS levels decrease as we age, so meditation could be nature's HRT.)

No. 25: Greater orderliness of brain functioning. (No more lost car keys.)

No. 34: Produces lasting beneficial changes in brain electrical activity. (Sparks will fly!)

No. 43: Improved learning ability and memory. (I *will* be able to succeed in all my challenges.)

No. 47: 'Mind ages at a slower speed'. (My main objective.)

* * *

I can't help but question if there is any scientific research that backs up these wonderful claims. So before I sign over my life to Belle's latest 'life-changing' scheme, I decide to consult my brain guru, Professor Simons. I send him the list and ask what he thinks. To my surprise — in common with most serious scientists he is a stickler for proven empirical evidence — his reaction is largely positive.

'I think most of the potential benefits mentioned are *possible*, but I don't know how many are backed by solid scientific evidence,' Professor Jon says. 'There's no doubt that meditation helps many people to feel better, focus more and build resistance to the everyday torrent of thoughts and anxieties.'

I tell him that the challenges I am undertaking — particularly the ones he has suggested might strengthen my cognitive skills, such as my French and music lessons — are making me a bit anxious. Would I benefit from this course?

'Being able to "clear" your mind so that you can focus your attention on the things that matter is obviously beneficial. And it could well have knock-on effects that fit with the potential benefits of meditation listed. If people feel those benefits, then it perhaps doesn't matter if that's due to a statistically significant mechanism or just due to the placebo effect,' he adds. 'Meditation is not going to harm anyone, so if someone feels the benefits of it then that's great. So yes, this could be really good for you, Jane.'

Week 1

With Professor Simons' blessing, I turn up full of hope the following Monday evening for the first of five lectures, given by the man Belle has nicknamed (in the nicest possible way) Magic Mike.

One of Belle's other BFFs, Laura, has generously offered to host the talks in her home (it's the kind of house that features in magazines like *Homes and Gardens* or *Architectural Digest*) and I am instantly overawed by and rather envious of my surroundings. The living room alone (which she calls 'the long room') is twice the size of my entire cottage. Still, I am determined not to let envy get between me and my spiritual well-being. Besides, the décor (cream sofas, soft lighting, candles, etc.) is as calming as it is sumptuous.

When we are sitting comfortably, Mike begins. There is something about him that justifies his nick-name (which has nothing to do with the film about a raunchy all-male dance troupe or the live stage show), even if, at first glance, he bears more resemblance to a jolly accountant than a spiritual guru. He describes himself as a 'Zen Buddhist, whose deep understanding has allowed him to bring self-realisation, knowing who and what one is, to a wide audience'.

Although this evening he has an audience of five – Belle, Ed (her husband), our hostess Laura, a woman called Annie, and me – he is so passionate about his subject and has such extraordinarily positive energy that within moments of my introduction to his method of meditation I am a believer. Mike tells us to sit upright, close our eyes and imagine an idyllic water scene – a beach or a lake in which we can see waves moving away from us (rather than, as they actually do, towards us). He tells us to count the waves in time with our in and out breaths and to visualise a number on each of those waves as they move away from us until we reach the tenth wave. I struggle with the direction of the waves but eventually summon up a lakeside scene that is perfect; and though I don't always see the numbers, it works for me. I am concentrating so hard, my overactive brain stops racing. We are to do this simple but effective meditation — repeated five times so that we see fifty waves — for approximately seven minutes, twice a day.

We then move on to Mindfulness, which involves 'slowing the pendulum of thought' by selecting two senses — your ears, eyes, touch, smell, etc. — and concentrating on what they perceive (in other words, focusing on what you are hearing and seeing, or what you can touch and smell) for five seconds. Mike explains that we should do this as often as we can in the day (he suggests every fifteen minutes) so that we can momentarily be in the *now*. As we progress, he informs us, we will be able to stay in the now for as long as five seconds. The ultimate goal, of course, is to always be in the now (reaching the state of enlightenment).

I mention to Mike that there are times when I feel I might be in a meditative state — or in the *now* — without realising it.

'I mean, I know its slightly shameful, but I love ironing because I don't think about anything other than what I am doing. Or things like peeling potatoes with a sharp knife — you can't do that and worry about the state of the nation, can you?'

He gives me a beatific smile (though I suspect he has already decided I am the problem pupil) and agrees that deep concentration on a particular task could be 'meditative', but perhaps peeling potatoes isn't the best option.

* * *

Back home, feeling ridiculously enthusiastic, I change my night-time routine. I abandon my usual bedtime reading (the Highway Code, my French textbook), turn off my iPhone and my iPad (on which I watch those French crime box-sets), and instead do a seven-minute meditation that sends me into a blissful sleep. My mornings are different too, beginning not with coffee but meditation. I religiously take time out during the day to try to be in the now. It's early days, but I am already feeling at least one of Mike's seventy-nine promised effects: No. 25: Greater orderliness of brain functioning.

Belle has set up a WhatsApp group for the five us, with a Buddha emoji and the title Buddha Babes (the only male in the class is Ed, Belle's husband, who has long since been considered an honorary Babe). The idea is that we can encourage each other and share any concerns we have, but — in the way that WhatsApp often does — our exchanges become the most entertaining part of our journey.

In the first few posts Laura, for example, reveals that she is finding it very hard to get in the 'now', while I'm having difficulty getting out of it; this prompts a flurry of responses asking how many potatoes am I peeling each day. Annie, the most logical and possibly intelligent person in our group, is finding it impossible to get her waves to roll away from her because this defies Newton's First Law of Motion — 'objects in motion will stay in motion unless acted upon by an outside force'. Annie has a degree in Physics, while I have an O level in Biology, so I don't argue with her. The fact that I can get my waves to go the way Mike has ordered is clearly another indication of my total inability to fathom the basics of science (although I do remember something about Newton and apples).

Week 2

By the time we are sitting down again in Laura's beautiful home, waiting for Mike to deliver our second lecture, we are Buddha-bonded. Which is a good thing because tonight's talk is seriously difficult. Mike attempts to convince us that nothing is solid, not even the sofas we are sitting on. Everything, he tells us, is energy, and our senses and minds create our world. He quotes Einstein: 'Everything is emptiness, form is condensed emptiness.'

If that wasn't tricky enough to grapple with, he moves on to talk about eradicating our egos, then ends by telling us the only place we can find reality is in our subconscious, which is not ruled by ego. To access our subconscious we have to reduce thought by silence and stillness. In the now (that is during the talk) I don't doubt a word Mike says, but I don't understand it either.

I may not have done all the homework he set in our first lecture (we were supposed to read three books which were out of stock on Amazon), but I have been doing my research. I have discovered Einstein's equation of

Ego and Knowledge — 'More the knowledge, lesser the ego; lesser the knowledge, more the ego'. While I accept that a lot of knowledge is a good thing, I am also aware that some of the best brains in the world have gigantic egos (Steve Jobs was renowned for his). I ask Mike if we would be where we are now (in Laura's amazing house with its state-of-the-art technology) if it wasn't for the human ego? He smiles and points out that in some ways that may be true, but the ego remains the biggest human problem and we will only find true happiness if we can transcend our ego.

I'm trying.

Week 3

In between the lectures the thing that seems to be bothering us all most on our WhatsApp group isn't anything to do with Einstein or 'Accepting that everything is emptiness'. No, it is how we are doing with our waves, which rather conveniently prompts our iPhones to produce an emoji of Hokusai's famous woodblock print *The Great Wave off Kanagawa*. Our other preoccupation is the Now (no emoji there) which is the place Belle and I have discovered our dogs seem to spend most of their time (either transfixed by a smell in the woods, or lying fast asleep with their legs in the air on the sofa).

When we mention our Zen dogs to Mike, he nods and informs us that all animals are in the now. They are not living in the past, worrying about what happened in the park last week, and they are definitely not living in the future because they are not encumbered with the kind of brain that is preoccupied with things like money, ambition or the ageing process.

He begins our session with a seven-minute group meditation and for the first time it works for Laura. It turns out that what had been holding her back was the association between waves and the riverside location of her house, which was dramatically flooded a few years ago. 'Every time I tried to visualise a wave, I saw the water overflowing from the river and coming to get me,' she tells us.

By now the rest of us have developed various methods of implementing our meditation — which we now call our fifty waves — into our lives. I do them in my morning bath and when I get into bed at night. Belle and Ed — who have one of those rare, ridiculously happy marriages — do them in tandem (they don't reveal where or when).

But we are all struggling with being in the *now*, although I have been pretty diligent about attempting it, if not every fifteen minutes, at least on the hour every hour (I have set my iPhone alarm to go off on repeat each hour during the day). This process produced an interesting reaction from my six-year-old granddaughter Edie when, during one of our regular Wednesdays together, the alarm went off as we were playing Sylvanian Families. 'What's that for?' she said. I tried to explain that the alarm was meant to remind me to take a minute out to go to the Now. 'Is that where the fairies live?' she asked me.

After our group meditation (and Laura's eureka moment), Mike is eager to move on to the next stage in our spiritual education. In my background research I have discovered that the 'essence of Zen Buddhism is achieving enlightenment by seeing one's original mind (or original nature) directly; without the intervention of the intellect'. And today's talk is about trying to work out 'what we are'. Mike informs us that we are not our body, our mind, our senses, our memory or our imagination, and we are absolutely *not* our egos — 'Learn to be detached and aloof and watch the antics of this terrible tyrant,' he warns us.

At the end of the talk, he challenges us to induce an out-of-body experience by trying to look down on ourselves as we are out doing something in our everyday lives. This experiment, he promises us, will prove what we really are (other than our body, mind, senses etc.).

Privately, I am beginning to wonder if Edie isn't right and all this 'in the now' business hasn't sent me 'away with the fairies'.

Week 4

The chat on our WhatsApp Buddha Babes group has slowed to the odd whisper. Only Annie has remembered to attempt the out-of-body homework that Magic Mike set us and reports that 'for a split second I really thought I was looking down on myself as I was walking home, but then I tripped on the pavement and I was back in my body and it hurt'.

We are, however, experiencing definite benefits from our Waves and our fleeting moments in the Now.

I am finding it much easier to focus on my other challenges, so it would seem that I am feeling the effect one of Mike's other promised 'benefits of meditation': 'No. 43: Improved learning ability and memory'. Plus I am sleeping better: 'No. 69: Requires less time to fall asleep, helps cure insomnia'. I am so calm that I may also be experiencing 'No. 47: Mind ages at a slower speed'.

Our penultimate talk, though, is tricky. Magic Mike tells us that 'the universe is a huge ball of energy, all is one' and that time doesn't exist — only the Now is real, the past and the future are all in our minds.

I am, as always, completely mesmerised by Mike; he is brilliant and inspiring and has so much goodness in him that questioning anything he says is almost impossible. But I worry about the idea he puts forward that language drives us away from 'the truth of oneness'. Mike tells us that when we 'don't cover the world with words, truth shines through'.

I tell Mike that I find it difficult to imagine a world in which human beings don't communicate with one another. 'Isn't "oneness",' I nervously say, 'a little self-obsessed and, er, selfish?'

He gives me another beatific smile and enthusiastically says, 'That's an interesting question, Jane.' But he doesn't give me a convincing answer and my inner journalist still believes that covering the world with truthful words can be a very positive thing. Particularly a world in which

Donald Trump, who dismisses any truth that doesn't benefit him as 'fake news', is the most powerful man.

Despite my occasional moments of scepticism, I am sure that much of what Mike is teaching us is working. Particularly his Mushin mantra that we learn at the end of our fourth lecture. His method of achieving what translates from the Japanese as 'no mind' involves closing your eyes and saying 'Mu' (Moo for us) on an outward breath and 'shin' on an inward breath, ten times in a row. By doing this it's possible to calm the mind at any tricky or irritating moment during the average day and it absolutely works for me. In the *now*, and I hope, in the forever.

Week 5

Since this is to be our final talk we have decided that irrespective of Magic Mike's rejection of materialism (he insists on giving the talks for free), we would all like to give him something, if only to cover his expenses for his trips to Laura's house. Belle buys a card (with a picture of Buddha) and we each sign it and put in £20.

I have to say, in fact we all have to say, that we feel a bit mean about how little we are paying for learning so much. But we don't want to offend him and the word is (from a previous group of Mike converts) that he would be horrified if we were to increase the amount.

Our final talk is very much a recap of everything we should have learned by now: reminding us that the goal is to eliminate what we are not — our bodies, minds, senses, memories — and concentrate instead on the Ocean of Awareness. If we are to find our real self we have to accept that we are not a person, we are aware-ness. If we allow our egos to dissolve, we will find the joy, bliss, peace and happiness that is our true self.

This heart-warming message makes us feel a little sentimental and emotional.

But then Mike gets rather serious and says that, although we might find it difficult, to be truly in a state of awareness, of oneness with the universe, we should make a pledge to never harm (let alone eat) any 'sentient beings'. The Buddhist definition of a sentient being is anything that is composed of five skandhas — matter, sensation, perception, mental formations and consciousness.

As we are all a little confused as to what this means, we get into a discussion about whether plants and trees might qualify as sentient. This, it turns out, is a grey area. Peter Wohlleben, in his book *The Hidden Life of Trees*, asserts that they are 'wonderful beings' and there is growing interest in the idea that plants are capable of 'intelligent behaviour'.

Magic Mike tells us that ideally we should start to follow a basic vegan diet and never knowingly harm or kill a sentient being (although he gives us the go-ahead to keep eating our greens).

I find myself confessing to the serial killing of at least a hundred bluebottles over the last few years, and Laura admits that she recently paid a pest control company to get rid of squirrels in her roof.

'In a perfect world,' Magic Mike responds, 'we should respect every living thing — even wasps, red ants and rats.'

Coming to terms with treating creepy-crawlies with respect is one thing, but not using or eating anything that contains animal products is quite another.

Like many people these days, the Buddha Babes rarely eat red meat but we all love chicken and fish and giving up all animal products maybe the hardest part of our lessons in meditation and mindfulness. Mike tells us that the popularity of veganism is not just about 'respecting every living thing' it is also about respecting ourselves (it's healthier) and respecting the environment (livestock contributes 18 per cent of human greenhouse gas emissions worldwide).

If we need convincing, he tells us to watch some of the recent documentaries *Dominion* and *The Game Changers* that support the argument for veganism.

I ask Magic Mike about alcohol because, while I think I can cope with becoming vegan, I am not sure (none of us are) that we can give up the odd glass of wine or G & T. But the fifth precept of a practising Buddhist is 'do not take intoxicants'.

'There are no rules in Zen Buddhism. We don't say you cannot drink or you cannot take drugs or anything else that might take over your life and become an addiction — gambling or even shopping,' he says. 'But if you follow the eightfold path of Buddha — which, put simply, consists of eight practices: right vision, right effort, right thought, right speech, right concentration, right attitude, right livelihood and right mindfulness — your need for those things will naturally drop away. When you discover who and what you are and understand that the desire to drink or take drugs or whatever is ego-driven behaviour, you won't need those things any more,' Mike says.

While some of what Mike has tried to instil in us over the last five weeks has been difficult to understand — if time doesn't exist, for example, why do his talks last exactly an hour and a half? — there is no doubt his message is a positive one. Zen Buddhism, unlike so many religious/spiritual creeds, is in no way judgemental (alcohol is not a 'sin' and gin, he informs us, is vegan).

Whether or not we have gained all seventy-nine of his promised 'benefits' is debatable, but what I've learned the last five weeks has supported me in my bid to take control of the ageing process by, at the very least, helping me sleep and (No. 72) decreasing my 'restless thinking'.

8

LIFE DRAWING

In which I learn more than I want to about human anatomy . . .

There is scientific evidence that taking up arts and crafts in some form is helpful for the ageing brain. But, as I have already established in my attempt to master the recorder, I am not one of those people who is 'good with their hands'. And the idea of doing something like a pottery class never appealed to me, perhaps because two of my closest friends are amateur potters and over the years they have given me gifts that look like nothing on earth. Is it an ashtray? Is it an animal of some kind? Is it a bowl? Whatever it is meant to be — and some of them were, admittedly, 'abstract' — it is usually hideous and not much more advanced than the kind of clay models my children brought home from school when they were five years old.

In fact almost all the craft ideas I research — particularly those with the word *Seniors* affixed to them — such as basket weaving, pom-pom making or creating something with mosaics or macramé — seem to me to be luring me back into a second childhood I am not quite ready to embrace. I know that a lot of people love crafts and are able to make beautiful and useful objects from everyday items like jam-jars, matchboxes and empty cornflakes packets, but personally I was never a fan of *Blue Peter*.

Research in 2015 carried out by the Mayo Clinic in Minnesota on 256 people aged eighty-five suffering from Mild Cognitive Impairment (MCI), revealed that those who took up painting, drawing or sculpting lowered their risk of developing dementia by an astonishing 73 per cent.

Another study, at the University of Waterloo, Canada, in 2018, found that people who were asked to draw quick pictures of words in a list of everyday items showed much better recall of those words than people who were asked to write the words multiple times. They concluded that drawing objects stimulates the brain because it requires elaborating on the meaning of the word and translating the definition into a new form — a picture. Using two study groups — one made up of young adults and the other of older adults — they found that the older adults were significantly less able to remember words they had written down than the younger participants, but they were equal to them in their ability to remember words they had drawn. The research concluded that 'taken together the evidence demonstrates that drawing is a robust encoding strategy that can, and does, improve memory performance dramatically'.

The more I look into art, memory and longevity, the more it makes me believe that I need to add drawing to my list of challenges. Pablo Picasso is quoted as saying that 'art washes away from the soul the dust of everyday life', and clearly it worked for him because he was still painting hours before he died, aged ninety-one, in 1972. Even doodling, I discover, can aid our ability to focus, relieve stress, and improve productivity and memory.

I have vague memories of loving drawing as a child and vivid memories of my children spending hours expressing themselves through art. At a young age we are uninhibited in our creativity and we don't think about the possibility of our art being judged by anyone else. As parents, we are so proud of our children's creations (regardless of their skill) that we frame them, stick them on the fridge and often treasure them forever (I have put up a clutch of my children's old work on the walls of my granddaughter Edie's bedroom).

Looking back, I realise that what made me stop drawing was that moment during school art classes when I knew I was being judged — and was consequently judging myself — as 'not very good'. Week after week, the teacher would choose artwork to display on the wall of the studio from the same three or four pupils. Having their work recognised served to spur those special girls on to try harder, do better and believe that they had a talent for art. But for me — and I think for the majority of the class — never being chosen for praise in painting or picture-making eventually turned me off a form of artistic expression that I had previously enjoyed.

One lesson lives on in my memory, despite art classes being deemed an unimportant part of the academic curriculum, relegated, as I recall, to one hour every Wednesday afternoon. Our teacher (her name escapes me) challenged us that particular day to create a picture of a boat of some kind — anything from a dinghy to an ocean-going liner.

In the first half of that lesson, I somehow managed to gain the teacher's attention. Along with one or two other of the initial drawings, she commented that my impression of a ship's hull was 'interesting'. For a moment I thought that maybe I could do this thing; I could join the elite of '*special*' girls in the class who were considered worthy of having their art displayed.

Inevitably, I messed up. And by messed up, I mean that when I came to add colour and poster paint to my creation I was so over-excited that I went at that first outline of my hull as if I were Jackson Pollock, never mind Picasso. In my head, I had this idea of a massive steel-coloured ship, highlighted here and there with a touch of bright red, yellow and green on its deck. So I overloaded my brush with a huge dollop of black, in the process splashing the collar of my white uniform shirt. Undaunted, having roughly covered most of the hull in a kind of tie-dye-effect charcoal, I set to work on the sea. I dipped my brush, without first cleaning it, into a pot of the brilliant blue that I was planning for the waves, but again I overdid it and the still-dripping hull of the ship blurred into the blue of the ocean and, well, sank. But it got worse; in my attempt to, as it were, raise the *Titanic*, I set to brightening up that deck — not to mention my white shirt — with a series of bright-red lifebuoys.

It was at this moment that I became aware of the first snigger from one of the *'special'* girls who had just put the finishing touches on her picture-perfect yacht. By the time I had added huge yellowish-orange sun in the murky-white cloudy sky, the entire class had joined the collective hysterics at the sight of my (I like to think, *Turneresque*) painting.

Redder in the face than those lifebuoys, I thought I might recover some credibility by pretending I had made that mess on purpose to elicit a response from my classmates. After all, I had gained a reputation as class clown in a number of subjects. But while I may have convinced the girls that my chaotic creation that day was a way of raising a laugh, the teacher gave me detention and privately I was crushed by both humiliation and bitter disappointment. I couldn't *do* art.

I have held on to that conviction that art was not for me, and have never dared to expose my vulnerability in a group class in the intervening four (or is it five?) decades. No doubt my cowardice in failing to take up any kind of art or craft since my schooldays explains my ungrateful reaction to the gifts created for me by brave and generous friends on the potter's wheel. Indeed, even with all the scientific evidence I have uncovered about the positive benefits of artistic endeavours, I remain reluctant to enrol myself in a class.

I decide to call Professor Simons in the hope that he will give me the final encouragement I need to take the plunge. And, of course, he does.

He tells me that taking up an art class is a great idea because it will involve 'focused concentration and in-depth analysis that taxes and stretches a number of cognitive abilities'. If I pay attention to what I am doing, I will be able to improve — and sustain with prac-tice (that again) — my ability to concentrate for longer periods and become better at 'avoiding distraction'. This is very encouraging, because one of my many lifelong failings is being, as most of my teachers (if they are still alive) would concur, 'easily distracted' (a much-repeated comment on my end-of-term reports).

According to Professor Simons, the positive benefits of taking art classes won't end there.

'It will be calming, relaxing and creative for you, Jane. It will lift your mood, reduce your anxiety and be generally good for your health and well-being.'

Is there, I innocently ask him, any particular art form that could be especially beneficial?

'It's up to you what you choose, but I would go for the most challenging thing and that would be life drawing,' he responds.

'Life drawing?' I exclaim, blushing at the very thought.

Professor Simons goes on to explain that one of the advantages to the brain of doing something like life

151

drawing over, say, completing a sudoku every day, is that every subject you draw is a new challenge. Sudoku might challenge your brain when you first start, but as you progress it is not working different parts of your brain. To get those other parts of the brain sparking, you have to do something *new*.

'Every life drawing class you attend will represent a fresh test of your cognitive skills. It's perfect,' he tells me, although I am not convinced that what I need is detailed cognitive study of naked human bodies.

I remind myself, though, that at least life drawing doesn't involve colour, paints and brushes. Everything had been fine with my twelve-year-old picture of a ship's hull until I had been told to *colour* it in.

Which is how I came to find myself, on a bright summer evening, joining the Wokingham Life Drawing Society's drop-in class run by the artist Mick McNicholas. As I have already indicated, I am not a very brave person and am particularly nervous about doing things on my own (I can't even go to the cinema alone), but having failed to convince Belle to join me on this venture, I have to overcome my reservations and summon up the courage to go solo into the unknown: a large office conference room in a building on an industrial estate.

I have no idea what to expect — chiefly whether it will be a naked man or a naked woman — but I have come prepared. I managed to find, in the brilliant bargain shop B&M, an A3 Quality Artist sketchbook (RRP £6.99 B&M price £2.99), plus a pack of sketching pencils and a box of charcoal (charcoal, apparently, is ideal for life drawing because it involves a lot of light and shade).

I have also done some basic preparation by ordering from Amazon a book called *Beginner's Guide to Life Drawing* (Search Press £9.99) by artist (and writer) Eddie Armer, which comes with illustrated instructions that will take you from a 'simple pose' to the difficult task of drawing anatomically correct hands and feet. He maintains that 'there is no better way to train your hand, eye and brain co-ordination and develop your powers of observation than life drawing'.

For a few days ahead of my first class I have been working on the not-so-simple pose and discovered that achieving 'basic body proportions' involves calculating that seven heads 'fit into an erect figure' and the 'tips of the fingers dangle mid-way along the thigh when an arm is relaxed'. Armer suggests anchoring the figure by drawing a central vertical line down the page and a horizontal line halfway down the main line so that you have a grid to build on. This, I realise, is going to be harder than I thought. You are meant to calculate the proportions of each body by 'eye', and since I am unable to draw a straight line without a ruler, I cheat and take one with me, hidden in my pencil case.

Mick charges £12 for each two-hour session (with free tea and biscuits during the break). Some of the money will go to the life model, who, I discover when I arrive, happens today to be a woman (phew!).

I explain to Mick that I am writing a book in which I challenge myself to do things that, I hope, will help me to hold on to my cognitive abilities into old age.

'And this challenge is going to be hard for me because I can't draw,' I add.

Mick reacts to this statement by covering his face with his hands in an expression of sheer desperation.

'You're like a lot of people I come across,' he says. 'You say you can't draw, but what you don't realise is that you can't draw unless you *do* draw. You don't imagine you are going to sit down at a piano for the first time and play Beethoven, do you? You understand you have to practise, to learn, to work as hard as you would if you were learning a language or a musical instrument.'

I gulp at this because, of course, I am already learning a language *and* a musical instrument, and I had rather hoped that Life Drawing would be more, well, recreational.

Mick directs me to a circle of chairs that surround a makeshift stage, covered in various bits of fabric (a length of velvet, a pile of silk, and so on) that is lit from above by a large camera light. The effect, it has to be said, is a little seedy (and that's before the model arrives). Behind the chairs are the easels; some people have brought their own, but Mick has a few he lends out. The turnout today is about thirty people with a roughly equal male – female split.

I take a seat next to a friendly-looking American woman in her thirties called Julie. She is, apart from

Mick, the only person in the room prepared to talk to such an obvious beginner (everyone else is very serious and competitive about their work). Before the model (who is currently sitting alone at the other end of the room modestly dressed in a bathrobe and flip-flops) makes her way to the stage, Julie and I bond.

A psychotherapist married to a British property developer, Julie is delightfully relaxed about her work. So relaxed, she has rejected the regulation A3 sketchbook for a small blank-page notebook. She tells me she originally started coming because she mistakenly thought it was a still-life not a life drawing class.

'I was late arriving and I walked into the room expecting to see a bowl of fruit and a vase of flowers and there was this naked man on the stage standing full-frontal,' she tells me.

At this point, I am almost crying with laughter at the thought of Julie's reaction. But there's admiration too, because she not only stayed but has kept coming back.

While we've been talking, the model has taken the stage, minus her bathrobe and flip-flops. She is, Mick announces, 'Millie, one of our favourite models', and he signals her to strike her first pose (each session starts with four five-minute poses).

Millie (who is naked apart from big hoop earrings) is attractive, about thirty-five, slim and medium-height. For her first pose she raises both her arms behind her head, which is covered in so much thick curly hair that it's difficult to make out her face. By the time I have ruled my vertical and horizontal lines and worked out the ratio of her head to her body (remembering that 'seven heads fit into an erect figure'), the bell sounds to indicate she should move to another pose and I haven't drawn anything.

But I use my plan for the first pose to attempt the second — she is standing with her back to us — and when the bell sounds again I have drawn a headless body with a huge bottom and stick legs. It looks like the kind of thing my granddaughter might produce (well, the stick legs, not the bottom).

In the third five-minute pose I surprise myself by doing quite a good drawing of her head and her shoulders (the earrings look particularly realistic) but I don't get as far as her chest before the bell rings again. In the fourth and final pose — with her back to us in such a position that from the chair I am sitting on to the left of the stage, one breast is revealed at an odd angle to her arms — I manage a reasonable reproduction of her left shoulder, arm and that breast, but I don't have time to fit in the nipple.

Two, slightly less taxing, ten-minute poses follow, then a twenty-minute pose that gives me enough time to replicate something that looks vaguely like Millie (complete with nipples).

During the fifteen-minute break for tea, I nervously approach Millie (back in her robe and flip-flops) and begin an innocent chat that is really my attempt at understanding what it is like to be a life model. It turns out that she is 'a suburban housewife with two children' for whom modelling in the evenings is a way to earn some extra money while her husband babysits. Millie is charming and funny and very matter-of-fact about her part-time profession. Her husband is fine with it and she has never had a problem with the male life-drawers. Besides, she adds, she 'goes into the zone' during the poses.

Millie's relaxed attitude reassures me, so much so that in the final forty-five-minute pose — in which she is sitting cross-legged on a tangle of velvet and polyester — I manage to sketch her entire body. Julie and I both think we have done quite well when we glance at each other's sketchbooks, although we both need to work on improving hands and feet (in mine, Millie appears to have paws and flippers).

But when we get up and take in everyone else's drawings we are not so confident about what we have achieved. Still, Mick says my sketches are 'quite good for a beginner', and the interesting thing is that I have really enjoyed myself. As Professor Simons predicted, I was totally absorbed in what I was doing to the point where the time flew by and I didn't once find myself distracted by thoughts of anything other than the subject in front of me.

* * *

Each week Mick emails us all to let us know the name and gender of the life model. In Week 2 he introduces Sylvana, who looks more glamour than life drawing model. She arrives on the stage in a belted black mac and high heels, which she removes in situ in a way that makes me feel a little uncomfortable.

Sylvana is petite and perfect, with long dark hair, but there is something about her that worries me. Particularly as today the music — which is usually the kind you get in a spa to suggest ocean waves and spiritual calm — is a selection of songs such as 'The Girl from Ipanema' (you know the one: tall and lovely and when she passes everyone goes 'a-a-a-h.).

But she is clearly a dream to draw and, despite my anxiety, her poses are so interesting/challenging that I surprise myself by not only getting both nipples in the right place, but also drawing what almost resemble two human feet.

As Julie and I make our way out we stop to admire the vastly superior work of the easel artists (a few of whom are professional). One man, clearly very pleased with his work, has drawn an intricately detailed replica of Sylvana's body but has left her eerily faceless, which I find unnerving.

To be fair, Sylvana is the only female life model in the classes I attend who makes me feel uncomfortable and causes me to question whether for some people life drawing might be more about voyeurism than art.

Mick, while he acknowledges that it is probably true that the more attractive the model (in his pre-class email he usually includes a portrait of the subject) the bigger the male turnout will be, disagrees that life drawing is in any way voyeuristic.

'I think that people who have never done it, and don't understand how difficult it is to draw a figure from life, might dismiss it as a bit iffy. It's anything but iffy. It's constantly challenging because every body is different, every pose is different, every expression is different and then sometimes when a model makes a move — and you are seeing them from another angle — they can look like a completely different person. If you stick at it, if you work at it, life drawing will become addictive,' he says.

It isn't until my sixth week that I am confronted by what has worried me most about this whole life drawing business — male genitalia.

I have never been one of those women who find the naked male form beautiful (although I have to admit Michelangelo's *David* and Leonardo's *Vitruvian Man* look quite nice).

I think this might have something to with the fact that my first ever sighting of a real-life penis occurred, in unpleasant circumstances, when I was fourteen. As I was taking a shortcut home from school one day, a flasher jumped out at me and demanded, 'What do you think of that . . .?' Looking back, I wish I had fired back, 'Not a lot' or 'Put it away for goodness' sake,' but I was so traumatised that I couldn't speak for a week and only managed to tell my mother when I was forty.

When I arrive, and take my regular seat next to Julie, I am unaware that this week's model is called Dennis because I didn't open Mick's email.

So the sight of a *man*, sitting on a chair to the left of the stage wearing a kimono and slippers, comes as a shock.

It's clear, before he slips out of his kimono and kicks off his slippers, that Dennis is no *David* or *Vitruvian Man*. By which I mean that he is about 5' 5" (in his slippers), hairy (he has a beard that looks as if it goes right down his neck to become chest hair) with proportions best described as 'cuddly'. If he changed his kimono for a duffel coat, he'd be a dead ringer for Paddington Bear. Which is reassuring.

But as cuddly as Dennis is (even when posing as Rodin's *The Thinker*) I am nervous about catching his eye. Or worse, him catching my eye when he moves into a full-frontal position and I am sizing up his proportions ('seven heads fit into an erect figure'). Dennis, though, turns out to be the perfect introduction to life drawing a male model.

In most of his poses (he is very imaginative, using a lamp at one point as a prop and managing to stand on one leg for the entire twenty-minute pose) is it impossible to make out exactly what lies beneath his stomach.

During the tea break, Julie and I become rather alarmed when Dennis, back in his kimono, walks over to us with his iPhone to appraise our work. He takes a photograph of my impression of him standing with the lamp (covering both his stomach and his bits) and pronounces that he 'really likes it'. I conclude that this is because I have made him look as if has more hair (on his head) than he does in life, and it makes him look ten years younger (and a couple of inches taller).

It isn't until the last forty-five-minute pose that I finally encounter his genitalia — well, what looks as if it might be his penis (if I lean my head to the right a bit) when he is sitting down with his legs widely parted. Afterwards, I am proud of how well I have captured his likeness and relieved that I was able to represent his manhood with no more than a barely visible shaded squiggle.

When I get home, I take a photo of my work, and put it up on the family WhatsApp to reassure my children that the nude male subjects their mother is drawing are not overtly masculine or threatening. They have been horrified by this particular challenge (and the one about *sex*), so I decide to caption the picture with the comment (which I know my son will find funny) 'Where's Willy?'

* * *

I am, as Mick predicted, getting, if not quite addicted, then really keen on life drawing. It is genuinely improving my concentration and is one of those things that could sit alongside (for me at any rate) playing puzzles or ironing (I know, I know — this might sound very out of character) in that I lose myself in them so much that they have a meditative effect on me.

Now that I have conquered my fear of male models I am feeling far more confident. And as the weeks pass,

I am clearly improving. Mick says that he is amazed at how quickly some people progress and that, within a year, with enough work and practice, I could be as good as some of the near-professionals in the class.

'The Easel People?' I say, stunned at the notion of joining the smug semi-pros who still don't talk to me (or Julie).

Christine, the artist friend who originally put me in touch with Mick, calls me one day to ask how it's going and to suggest she might join me at the drop-in class that Monday. I find this a little daunting because her work — she specialises in portraiture — is brilliant, but I agree and we turn up knowing only that this evening's life model is new (so no portrait) and his name is Lorenzo.

We sit together (Julie is away) and we are talking so much that we don't pay much attention to what is happening on the stage until Mick announces that Lorenzo is ready to start, as usual, with four five-minute poses.

One of the important side effects of my life drawing classes has been discovering that every human body is different. Most of the models are female and in drawing them I have realised that their bodies are beautiful regardless of their age or their size, and this has been liberating. Like a lot of women, I have never been entirely happy about my body and life drawing has made me understand there is no such thing as the 'perfect female form', and worrying about weight (and gravity) as I grow older is self-destructive and silly. Moreover, I have discovered that there is no such thing as the 'perfect male form'; men come in as many different shapes and sizes as women.

But Lorenzo . . . suffice it to say that Christine gasps when she starts calculating his measurements and I am (unusually) lost for words. It's the very thing I have been dreading since starting these classes. Because there is no way of avoiding Lorenzo's genitalia. In the first four five-minute poses (even when he has his back to us) his manhood is visible. (To my horror, I realise his proportions work out as roughly 'seven penii fit into an erect figure').

What makes it all the worse is that Lorenzo is no more than thirty-five (most of the male models are at least forty-five) and facially does look rather like da Vinci's *Vitruvian Man* — with similar features and a matching mop of thick, long hair.

'I'm not sure I can do this,' I whisper to Christine.

'It's certainly challenging,' she replies.

While previous models have used props in some of their poses — draping velvet across their shoulders, using a cane to add interest or placing their hands in such a way that their bits are not the focus of attention — there is nothing in the room, apart from perhaps one of the easels, that could conceal Lorenzo's manhood. A fig leaf would be pointless.

In the twenty-minute pose before we break, I decide to focus away from the obvious and draw his fine head and wide shoulders.

During the interlude, to my relief Lorenzo wraps a towel around his waist to cover his lower body and sits down on a chair away from the rest of us to study his phone. Mick comes over to look at our work. Appraising Christine's brilliant reproduction of Lorenzo's body, he whispers, 'No one will ever believe you!' and the three of us struggle to control our laughter. (That night, I post a slightly edited version of my drawing on to our family WhatsApp, superimposing a cartoon whale over Lorenzo's manhood, with the caption 'Free Willy'.)

I have collected myself for the final forty-five-minute pose and I am determined to try to capture Lorenzo's image in its entirety (he is lying down with his arms supporting his head). And it is then that I realise how brilliant life drawing is, because I am so absorbed in the process that I stop thinking about anything other than — as Eddie Armer puts it — translating 'our complex three-dimensional world and to represent it two-dimensionally within the confines of a sheet of paper'.

In the process, I have overcome that fear of my drawings being judged, or of being, as I was back in school, mocked and humiliated. I no longer care what other people think of my work, and that's an incredibly positive step for me. I am now drawing simply for pleasure and relaxation, having banished the sense I am competing to belong to an elite group of the population who have been recognised as 'talented'. As Mick said to me at my first class, '*anyone* can draw'.

LIFE DRAWING

Another interesting thing about my life drawing classes is that it has taught me to properly observe people and see details I would never have noticed. Sometimes, when I am at the supermarket or maybe the cinema, I will see someone sitting or standing in an unusual position and find myself itching to grab my B & M Sketchbook and draw them (with their clothes on, obviously).

I am seeing the world from a totally different perspective and loving my classes so much that I am thinking of buying an easel.

9

THE MYSTERIES OF THE MACROBIOME

In which I attempt to Marie Kondo my gut . . .

It was Belle who first suggested it would be a good idea to look into ways of rejuvenating my innards along with the rest of me. Way ahead of the curve when it comes to beauty and body crazes, Belle is always coming up with amazing ideas that 'could be life-changing'. I think everyone has a friend like her — I call her *my* BFF, but the truth is everyone is Belle's BFF. She is hilarious, opinionated and brutally honest when necessary. But she is also the kind of person, as I have learned to my peril during the course of our friendship, to whom it would be impossible to say no.

Saying 'yes' to her (when I longed to say no) has taken me on some strange adventures, usually as research for an item for her online magazine. The highlights of which, looking back, have probably been a Burlesque lesson (with costumes), a Colonic Cleansing session in a seedy London spa, and our paddle-boarding course (she elegantly floated, I sank).

But the truth is that this time I owe her not just because she gamely joined me in my bid to master the recorder and bravely came with me to learn about G-spots and glow-in-the-dark dildos but also because she coerced me into doing things I didn't want to that turned out to be precisely what I needed (such as ballroom dancing). It's almost as if Belle knows what is good for me in a way I don't. On that basis, I agree to embark on a twenty-one-day Macrobiome Purify Programme devised by a company called Synergy, despite having no idea what it might entail and not being able to afford it (at £202 for the three-week kit!).

'If you follow this programme with me you will have the digestive tract of a twelve-year-old. It will boost your mental health and your immunity,' she assured me one day in late February, the time of year at which most of us are feeling bloated and blue.

After I have paid, I read up on the origins of Synergy and discover that, while their products are marketed as pure, organic and 100 per cent 'made in the USA', their international headquarters are in Spain. The products are sold through 'Synergy Elite Health Advisors' (ours is a friend of Belle's) who earn a basic commission of 10 per cent by finding new clients who will become regular returning customers (like an upmarket Avon Lady).

I justify the expense to myself because it will be good research for this book. Apparently, achieving the right balance of bacteria, fungi and microflora in my micro-biome can rejuvenate the ageing gut. After three weeks on this regime (according to the exhaustive information given to us by our 'Elite Health Advisor'), Belle and I will emerge as happier, healthier, more energetic and, by the way, slightly slimmer people. I am ashamed to admit that, despite my support of the Body Positivity movement, this last effect (weight loss) did play a part in my decision to go ahead with the programme. I am not very tall, have a small frame and normally weigh about 8½ to 9 stone, but over the winter I have moved closer to 10 stone (i.e. 9 stone 13 pounds)

Putting vanity aside, I don't go totally blindly into the regime. My initial research into the gut microbiome, merely scratching the surface of Google, is mind-blowing. Since time began (well around the late fourth and early third century BC), the idea of the gut being vital to good health was being mooted (it was Hippocrates who said 'all disease begins in the gut'). We now know that the human body contains around ten times as many microbes, most of them in the gut, as it does human cells (which, I presume, means that we are more microbe than human).

The microbiome is a vast ecosystem of organisms — bacteria, yeasts, fungi, viruses and protozoans — that live in our gut. Collectively, these organisms weigh up to a kilogram (heavier than the average brain), and scientists are beginning to treat the gut microbiome as an organ in its own right. Each gut contains around 100 trillion bacteria, many of which are essential in breaking down food and toxins, making vitamins and building up our immune systems (80 per cent of the immune system lives in our gut).

As we age, we tend to have less varied types of gut bacteria, which makes our digestive systems weaker than that of younger people so, in theory, following a diet that involves boosting the amount and variety of bacteria in my gut will have a positive effect on my health. Since 90 per cent of serotonin (which is supposed to make us feel a natural high) is also produced in the gut, there is every reason to suppose I will feel happier after my three-week programme.

It would seem, though, that gut cleansing/balancing via a bewildering array of products and programmes is a multibillion-dollar business worldwide. The company I have signed up to has hundreds of competitors offering similar promises of improved health. Chuckling Goat, Microbiotica, Symprove are among those making claims about the cure-all effects of balancing the gut. Conditions as varied as IBS, type 2 diabetes, depression and arthritis are among those said to benefit. Most of these companies are dismissive of well-known brands of probiotic-drinks and yogurts that fill the shelves of supermarkets, insisting that few of them − as they promise their particular products *do* − reach the gut as live bacteria.

This notion of good bacteria reaching our gut alive and being able to 'set up home' and colonise is regarded as key to changing and improving our inner ecosystem. Achieving this goal is a challenge, because in order to make it to the intestine, the probiotics must pass through the stomach, which is a hostile acidic environment that can kill beneficial bacteria.

As difficult and confusing as it is to wade through the often-conflicting promises made by both the branded supermarket probiotic products and the more comprehensive (and expensive) microbiome-boosting regimes on the market, I decide to throw myself into the Synergy programme. It is, anyway, too late to back out now (since I won't get my money back).

Besides, all I have to do in the first week is cut out alcohol, caffeine, dairy, sugar, starch, wheat and 'all processed foods', drink two litres of water a day and take two 'Body Prime' capsules (a magnesium-based supplement) every morning to prepare my body for what is to come and to reduce cravings. This is, of course, easier said than done, since most days for me start with three cups of coffee, and quite a few of them end with two glasses of red wine. Belle and I decide to begin our twenty-one-day programme at Lent, symbolically starting on Ash Wednesday on the basis that we might need God on our side.

Our Synergy Elite Health Advisor has set up a WhatsApp group called Microbiome Purify for March on which we can communicate with each other and ask her any questions we might have. So here goes.

Day 1: Wednesday, 6 March 2019

Last night I did that thing that I haven't done since I was about twenty-four — I consumed everything forbidden that was left in my fridge, my freezer and my wine rack.

Well, it was Pancake Day (or Fat Tuesday, as it is also known), and the prospect of three weeks' deprivation gave me a reasonable excuse to pig out. In the space of around three hours I ate four chicken thighs, a bag of oven chips, a whole carton of Ben & Jerry's Chunky Monkey ice cream, three packets of Mini Cheddars and four pancakes topped with maple syrup. Oh, and an entire bottle of red wine.

The only positive aspect of this disgusting indulgence is that I was feeling so sick and intoxicated when I went to bed that detoxifying was the only way forward today. I am not sure whether ibuprofen is allowed, and I know black coffee definitely isn't, but the two litres of fizzy water I drink helps a bit.

Day 3: Friday, 8 March

I am doing OK eating what they call microbiome-friendly foods that contain the prebiotic inulin: leeks, onions, chicory, blueberries, beans, cold potatoes and lots of garlic. Fermented foods are high on the list, too, and I have a strange liking for sauerkraut, but all in all it isn't much fun.

Our Synergy Elite Heath Advisor puts up some 'delish' recipes on the WhatsApp group including 'Fish and Chips!', but when this turns out to be a small piece of grilled cod in oat crumb with a meagre portion of sweet potato fries and broccoli, I don't bother.

The worst thing, for me, is that I am suffering from the kind of caffeine withdrawal symptoms I would have expected if I were coming off heroin (think *Trainspotting*). I have a permanent headache, can't sleep and feel nauseous most of the time. Belle, meanwhile, is sailing through the first week. She is devouring the WhatsApp micro-biome recipes and is baffled as to why I am experiencing anything other than a 'feeling of contentment'.

Day 5: Sunday, 10 March

I am still waiting for Belle's 'feeling of contentment' to arrive. So far, having existed for the last five days on a diet of fermented foods, raw vegetables and lentils, I have a gut feeling that is anything but *content*. In fact, I feel like a human whoopee cushion, so full of accumu-lated gas and air that I am a danger to public health. So over-inflated, indeed, that just embarking on a trip to the supermarket has become a problem, lest I find myself taking off in the vegetable aisle of Sainsbury's.

Against the odds (and all the wind) I seem to be constipated.

Our Elite Health Advisor assures me that this 'will pass, literally!' and adds cheerily, 'When you finally do go, it feels almost like colonic irrigation!'

On the plus side, I have 'come off' caffeine (and red wine).

Day 6: Monday, 11 March

This is the day when the hard work begins. For the next week Belle and I are to follow what the manufacturers call a 'carefully engineered programme of clinically formulated supplements: Biome Shake, DT, Biome Actives, Body Prime, ProArgi-9'. The ingredients for all these magical supplements are 'ethically and organically' sourced from peas, broccoli, chicory root, flaxseed, rice bran, cabbage, carrot, black bean, adzuki bean, turmeric, borage and 'many more'. All topped up by the addition of every vitamin, mineral and amino acid you can name (and an awful lot you can't). YUM!

I start the day with my regular two Body Prime capsules followed by new Biome Active capsules. These combine Bacillus coaglulans — good bacteria — with inulin, a fibre found in foods such as chicory and garlic, which encourages the development of this good bacteria and discourages bad bacteria. Then it is almost time for my breakfast proper — two scoops of powdered Biome shake packed with yet more things I have never heard of, listed in detail (that I won't bore you with), which I mix with water in my Breville Blend-Active Pro Blender (half the price of a Nutribullet).

Mid-morning and mid-afternoon I mix two sachets of Biome DT with water, hold my nose, and drink (it tastes disgusting), plus one sachet of ProArgi-9 (sweeter and fruitier) also mixed with water. I am allowed a 'snack' of nuts, fruit or oatcakes but pass on this so-called 'treat' because, frankly, I need something closer to a Krispy Kreme Doughnut.

By lunchtime I am not so much hungry as exhausted — I find reading instructions taxing and getting the right product at the right time has killed my appetite. But I force myself to gulp down another Biome shake.

I choose my evening meal (which they suggest I eat before 8 p.m.) from the list of biome-friendly foods that I ate in Week 1. They recommend a lot of legumes (soya beans, dried beans, lentils and chickpeas), some protein (fish, nuts, etc.) and some fruit.

Thankfully, I have finally had what my mother used to call a 'movement', only this one has a magnitude that equates to 7 on the Richter scale. Indeed, from now on, I have been warned it is unwise to wander more than fifty yards from a 'facility' (i.e. a toilet) and to stay well downwind of anyone you love. Even Zorro, the kind of dog that follows you everywhere, is beginning to avoid me.

Day 9: Thursday, 14 March

On the way back from a work meeting in London, I am suddenly overwhelmed by a feeling of urgency that I can only compare to the final stage of labour. The traffic is gridlocked and there are no 'facilities' between my car and my downstairs loo at home (about fifteen miles away). Rather like the nursery rhyme I was taught at antenatal classes to repeat again and again during contractions, I find myself using Magic Mike's Moo-shin mantra. An intake of breath on the 'Moo' and an outtake on the 'Shin'. I don't stop after ten (the point at which your mind calms) and carry on until I get home and make it, just in time, to the loo.

(Thanks, Magic Mike.)

Day 11: Saturday, 16 March

Some time ago I had put 'babysitting Edie' in my diary for tonight, and since my daughter has an important function to attend I cannot back out. The nights I spend with my granddaughter in London involve a very set routine. We go out to her favourite restaurant — a branch of Byron's in Clapham — eat everything Mummy doesn't usually allow, and then go home and have what we call our Happy Hour. This involves us watching a movie in our pyjamas while we feast on a variety of forbidden snacks (Pringles, pickled-onion-flavoured Monster Munches, Pomme Bears and Cinema Sweet popcorn) and our favourite drinks (apple juice for Edie, red wine for Granny Annie).

But this is the last day of the intensive part of my three-week programme and I dare not stray from the regime. Not just because it has cost me so much (physically and financially), but also because Belle (who is feeling 'absolutely brilliant' and doesn't understand why I am 'making such a fuss') would kill me. Her journey to gut health has been so much easier than mine, involving almost no caffeine/alcohol withdrawal symptoms and none of my unwelcome digestive problems. This, I suspect, is because she is naturally very disciplined and is not the kind of person who would ever have a supper consisting entirely of Kettle Chips and Chianti. With Belle in mind, I summon up the self-control to resist a double burger (with extra cheese, bacon and fries) when Edie and I go to Byron, and opt instead for a salad with no dressing. Back home, buoyed up by this restraint, I am also able to watch, rather than partake, while Edie enjoys Happy Hour.

In the morning Bryony – who is eighteen months into sobriety – gives me some of the tips she has picked up for filling in the time that you would normally be eating (in my case) or drinking (in her case). These include having body massages at home in the evening, enjoying long candlelit pampering baths and going to bed early with her husband/and or a good book. Back home that night I implement some of her suggestions. I have a long candlelit bath and am in bed with a good book by 9.20, feeling a little sad about not having a husband too.

Day 15: Wednesday, 20 March

A curious thing happens today. I am on a long and windy country walk with the dog when I experience a moment of extraordinary elation. In other words, I feel – for no other reason I can think of apart from my beautifully balanced macrobiome – ridiculously *happy*.

This must be the 'feeling of contentment' that Belle has been enjoying since Day 2 of our regime. At last, I can see the point of this whole dreary business. Although since Monday I am over the worst and am back on three healthy (i.e. dull but gut-friendly) meals a day (plus a shake, my capsules and one of the nicer-tasting supplements), it seems that, finally, the process is working. As a result, I am becoming a microbiome bore — telling everyone I come across (even the postman) about the poisons that we unwittingly throw down our digestive tracts ('I am at one with my gut now,' I mutter).

Day 18: Saturday, 23 March

As I near the end of the programme, I smugly assure myself that I have conquered all those cravings for *bad* foods and that I will be able to live on this programme for the rest of my (long and healthy) life. I might get older, but my gut will be younger than springtime. I start reading up on the maintain-your-microbiome after-programme. Rather flatteringly, my Synergy Elite Health Advisor says that she would like to make me a *VIP* customer with privileges such as a discount when I re-order products (presumably for the rest of my long and healthy life).

I am so obsessive about my new way of living that I have convinced myself the craving for coffee first thing in the morning and a packet (or two) of Red Leicester Mini Cheddars with my glass (or two) of red wine in the evening was a devilish psychological reward system I had set up which had turned into a self-destructive habit. I had even come to believe that those 'treats' tasted as disgusting as that first glass of Biome DT I drank back on Day 6. By now, Biome DT — made of psyllium husk, glutamine, cabbage leaf, carrot root and chicory root — seems more delicious to me than cheese straws and a bottle of Merlot.

Day 21: Tuesday, 26 March

This, the final day of the three-week programme, is the moment I have decided to finally stand on the scales. Belle has been weighing herself every day and has lost 11 pounds, but I had held back for today's big reveal. While I don't think I have lost more than 7 pounds, I am looking forward to seeing the benefits of everything I've put myself through in the last twenty or so days.

But, you guessed it, when I climb on to my digital scales (wearing nothing, not even my watch and glasses) I discover that I weigh 9 stone 11 pounds. I have lost exactly 2 pounds. I am so disappointed about this particular aspect of my marvellous new regime that I talk to our Health Advisor, who reassures me: 'For a lot of people, the weight falls off several weeks after they have finished the initial programme and are on the maintenance plan.' I transfer £132.50 (that I don't have) to her for the first month of the after-programme.

Day 24: Friday, 29 March

Perhaps if I hadn't had such a stressful day (I think Mercury must be in retrograde), I wouldn't have ended my macrobiome experience in rather the way I had started it (back on Fat Tuesday).

Driving back from London in appalling weather and particularly bad Friday-night traffic, I can't stop thinking about *real* food. My meal for tonight (a cold steamed salmon steak and some kale) is in the fridge waiting for me, but all I can think about is big slices of bread smothered in butter and topped with full-fat cheese and sweet pickle; triple-cooked chips dipped in mayonnaise; roast potatoes and Yorkshire puddings; scones with strawberry jam and clotted cream.

It's almost 10 p.m. when I finally reach my local town centre (where most of the shops are shut by 5 p.m.) but, miraculously, there is a free parking space outside the late-night Sainsbury's Local and I push my way through the automatic doors in a murderous mood. I buy the shop.

At home I feverishly feast on my poisonous purchases (Kettle crisps! Cheddars! Belgian buns! Minstrels!) washing them down with two, three, four glasses of Malbec. Then I eat the big Lindt bunny that I had bought as an Easter treat for Edie, and suddenly remember that there are three of her Nobbly-Bobbly ice lollies still in the freezer.

By 11.30 p.m. I am in sugar and alcohol shock. Never mind 'the feeling of contentment' I got from my beautifully balanced microbiome, I am now experiencing the kind of extreme joy you get from junk food and a flagon of red wine.

At least I am for the half an hour it takes me to stumble up the stairs, slip into bed and fall asleep. In the morning, horribly hungover, I call Belle to confess my fall from gut grace. But before I can list my 'sins', she interrupts me.

'I cheated last night,' she says in a regretful voice. 'I grated some parmesan over my cabbage greens.'

I say nothing.

* * *

For the next week I try my best to get back on the Microbiome track, but the spell is broken. I have remembered that the taste of Red Leicester Mini Cheddars, particularly when accompanied by a glass of red wine, is totally delicious and that nothing, certainly not Biome DT, tastes as wonderful as a packet of chocolate Minstrels.

I would probably have given up on the positive effects of good bacteria on my gut altogether if I hadn't been commissioned, a couple of weeks later, to write a feature − and undergo an accompanying photo shoot − with the worrying brief: 'Can a woman look sexy over the age of fifty?'.

Since I was now back to my winter weight (just under 10 stone) and the last time I had done a photo shoot for the *Telegraph*'s *Stella* magazine I had been at my summer low of 8 stone 7 pounds, I decided that I had to do something, and fast. Fast, as it turns out, being the operative word. As far back as it's possible to go, fasting has been linked to good mental and physical health. (Plato declared, 'I fast for greater physical and mental efficiency.') In today's world — in the fight against obesity — there is growing interest in limiting our energy intake via regimes such as intermittent fasting. The mad, bad and maybe dangerous diets of the past that were often contradictory (high fat, low fat, fibre only, etc.) have given way to programmes that lower the total intake of food via alternating periods of fasting and eating, such as the 5:2 method (fasting two days and eating five) and 16:8 (fasting for sixteen hours a day and eating in a window of eight hours).

When I had first been researching gut health I had come across a company called Nosh Detox that did a range of organic products to 'purify the body inside and out'. If I were to do their six-day Juice Fast I would, Geeta Sidhu-Robb (who founded the company) told me, lose at least 5 pounds and would also feel radiant and look terrific. It was going to cost me (£331) and push me further into the overdraft, but friends who had previously done the fast assured me it was worth it.

Each day of the fast I will start with a ginger-and-lemon tonic as soon as I wake up and will then have four (500 ml) bottles of Raw, fresh, unprocessed, naturally blended juices that I will drink at 11 a.m., 1 p.m., 4 p.m. and 8 p.m. The first two days' supply arrives on my doorstep packed in ice and sealed in a polystyrene box.

Drinking the ginger-and-lemon tonic — which is very sour — is difficult, but the juices themselves are delicious. Each one is blended with different fruits and

vegetables relevant to the time of day you have them
— to boost your energy during the working day and to
relax you in the evening. I don't have any hunger pangs
— not just because each bottle is filling, but because I
have emptied the house of anything I could possibly
eat were I to feel tempted (apart from the dog and cat
food, and I am fairly confident I won't sink that low).

By the time the second box arrives, for days 3 and 4,
I am a committed fan and already experiencing some
of the promised health benefits (I am, though, quite
suggestible, so it's possibly all in my head rather than
my gut). I am, too, feeling more confident about my
forthcoming photo shoot, despite an email from the
stylist asking for my bra size as she has 'found some
fabulous sophisticated but super-sexy lingerie'.

On Day 7 (the day of the shoot) I discover I have
lost 9 pounds on the fast and am now weighing in at
9 stone 4 pounds. I am still, though, concerned about
the clothes the stylist has assembled because I told her
I was a size 10 when I am a size 12/14.

I don't know whether it is the encouragement of
the photographer, the artful way the make-up artist
has made me up or the general light-headedness that
comes from going without solid food for six days, but
I feel marvellous. In fact, almost sexy. The pictures are
ridiculously flattering (there is clearly Vaseline on the
camera lens or some serious photoshopping is going on)
and although I feel a bit faint by 3 p.m. (these sessions
take forever), I am happy at the end of the long, long day.

It has to be said that I undertook both these regimes motivated as much out of vanity as concerns for my health, but I genuinely felt well on them. I had more energy, I felt positive, focused and found it easier to sleep. But I do question the idea of a permanently restricted diet. Surely one of life's greatest pleasures is the occasional indulgence in those things that are not necessarily microbiome-friendly?

What's more, both the programmes were extremely expensive. If you have the time, it's possible to create your own gut-cleansing regime using fresh organic fruit and vegetables. There are hundreds of DIY gut-supporting ideas online that you can implement (although it's best to check with your doctor before embarking on a home-made regime). For example, a DIY Water Flush, involving drinking six to eight glasses of lukewarm water a day and eating foods with a high water content (watermelons, tomatoes, strawberries, cucumber, lettuce) is possibly as effective as my six-day juice fast. As is upping your intake of probiotic-rich fermented foods — yogurt, kefir, pickles, kombucha and miso. Resistant starches — potatoes, rice, legumes, green bananas and grains — are also good for naturally boosting your gut microflora.

But I am still not entirely convinced that the gut is the holy grail of good health. So it's time to seek an expert opinion as to whether this is a passing fad (fuelling a probiotic industry expected to be worth £48 billion by 2023) or sound science.

John Cryan, Professor and Chair at the Department of Anatomy and Neuroscience at University College Cork, believes that with further advances in the field it may be possible to diagnose brain diseases and mental health problems by analysing gut bacteria. By introducing specific bacteria, dubbed 'psychobiotics', to the microbiome, they hope that in the next few years they will be able to successfully treat, or at least help, some of these conditions. I tell him about my efforts at gut cleansing, and ask whether he believes such programmes can help us as we age.

'The microbiome is like a rainforest in that it is a whole ecosystem within us, and we know that diversity is very, very important. But it is early days, and we are not there yet. There is hope, but we haven't even identified exactly what constitutes a normal microbiome,' he says.

At this point I feel impelled to let Professor Cryan know that my science credentials are limited to the O level in Human Biology I took when I was sixteen.

'A lot of these companies who are making a lot of money out of selling products that supposedly support gut health tend to make extraordinary claims for which, in my opinion, they have insufficient scientific evidence. Regulation in this area should be improved, particularly in the United States, where they can say anything without full or widespread back-up research. A lot of it could just be snake oil,' he says.

In defence of my twenty-one-day programme, I tell him about the sense of elation I experienced at the end of the second week, and how the only thing I could attribute it to was my newly balanced microbiome.

'What were you doing when this feeling overwhelmed you?' he asks me.

'I was walking the dog,' I reply.

'That explains it!' shouts Professor Cryan. 'We know that dogs and green spaces are beneficial to the micro-biome. It was probably more to do with your dog and your environment than your diet.'

Apparently Zorro is as good for my gut as sauerkraut, because he brings into my home such a varied amount of bacteria that my 'indoor microbiome' (the billions of bacteria, viruses and fungi in homes and workplaces) exposes me to more diverse bacteria than my cat, and a great deal more than very house-proud folk without a pet will experience.

Professor Cryan in no way dismisses the benefits of a diet rich in fresh fruit, vegetables and fermented foods, but he questions the 'added value' of processed supplements.

'Some of these products have outrageous claims about health benefits that are not backed up by sound evidence and should have a "buyer beware" sticker on them. It's questionable how much good they do, but then again I doubt any of them will do you real harm,' he says.

In Professor Cryan's view, the best programme I could follow would be the Mediterranean Diet — based on the traditional healthy foods consumed by people from countries bordering the Mediterranean Sea. Although this varies from country to country (France, Italy, Spain) the main ingredients are very similar. They all have a high content of vegetables, fruit, legumes, nuts, beans, cereal, grains and unsaturated fats such as olive oil, and a low intake of meat, sugar and dairy products.

'Research has consistently shown that if you follow such a diet it will lower your risk of developing cardio-vascular diseases and overall mortality,' Professor Cryan adds.

I ask him something that has been worrying me since I started on this particular journey: the fact that we are made up of ten times more microbes than human cells.

'Are we human or are we microbes?' I ask him (with apologies to The Killers and their song 'Are We Human or Are We Dance?').

'For years people have been using that phrase "we are what we eat",' Professor Cryan replies. 'In reality, we are what our microbes eat.'

I have taken Professor Cryan's advice and while I've been embarking on other challenges I have been eating Mediterranean and microbiome-friendly meals to support my health and help me maintain high energy levels. One of the most interesting – and perhaps positive – side effects of paying attention to (as Professor Cryan puts it) 'what my microbes eat', is that on the (now very rare) occasions when I do indulge in high-fat/processed/sugary foods, I feel sick and lethargic.

But the most heartening (figuratively and literally) thing I have discovered, thanks to Professor Cryan, is that one of the best ways of encouraging the growth of good bacteria and, at the same time, inhibiting the development of bad bacteria in your gut is to consume foods that contain polyphenols. These are plant-based micro-nutrients that are full of health-giving antioxidants. And guess what? The stilbene polyphenol, resveratrol, contained in red wine is not only believed to be good for your gut, but also for your brain and your heart.

Sadly, there are no such health benefits in Red Leicester Mini Cheddars or chocolate Minstrels.

10

ENDURANCE, STRENGTH, BALANCE AND FLEXIBILITY

In which I overcome my fear of the gym and learn to love squats, weights and punchbags . . .

From the start I knew that I would have to take on a serious fitness challenge for this book. Friends who know about my fear of gyms and indeed any sweat-inducing, heart-thumping exertion of any kind suggested I do something gentler, such as yoga (which I know does get tough as you progress) or Tai Chi (said to be excellent for the elderly). But I knew if I was going to be true to the aim of *How Not to Get Old*, I had to do something that would have a positive effect on my physical fitness that could also be *proven*.

But there are gyms and there are gyms, and looking for the right one took a while. I eventually made an appointment at a highly recommended establishment run by a woman who was very inspiring; she was around my age, looked amazing and was passionate and knowledgeable about supplements, diet, hormones and health. I told her about the aim of my book, confessed that I had never exercised and that, because of my deadline, I had a maximum of five months in which she could 'turn me round'. She looked at me and shook her head saying that with my poor muscle tone, worrying BMI (whatever that was) and general lack of fitness, it would take a year to 'get anywhere'.

We talked for a while and she finally said that she would take me on but that it would involve so much of her time (and mine, since she wanted me to work out with her at least six times a week) that I would have to pay a substantial sum of money in advance. It has to be said when the amount was mentioned (£2,000) I was a little alarmed, but by then I felt like Mowgli in the *Jungle Book* when he was hypnotised by Kaa the snake, entreating him to 'trust in me'.

As I have already established, I am very suggestible, and I found myself mesmerised by everything she had to say. So much so that I was in the process of mentally drafting a request for a bank loan to cover the cost, when she suddenly started talking about the things I could do to make my face look younger. She would put me on to a doctor who did an amazing 'peel'; she could recommend someone who could give me an 'eye lift'; and she was certain that those 'little lines above your lips' could be treated.

I realised then that she had not understood the aim of my book, which was not about looking younger and having cosmetic surgery — something that strikes me as

dangerous and decadent — but about undertaking challenges that would sharpen my brain and build up my
body in order to protect myself for the onward march
to old age. Coward that I am, I didn't exactly turn her
down but said I would get back to her — then left,
never to return.

But the other big — and obviously much cheaper
— gym chains didn't attract me either because of their
size and the fact that there seemed to be an unstated
membership age limit of twenty-five.

Looking back, I can't help but feel that some kind of
magic led me to the door of a small specialist gym that
I happened to drive past one day. Because I am not sure
I could have completed this challenge without Ash, the
manager of Fitness Space, who I met that day in June
and who persuaded me that he could turn me into a
gym bunny in five months for a bargain rate that would
include a full year's membership (£450) as well as ten
sessions with him as my personal trainer.

Ash was astonished that I was a 'gym virgin'. I told
him that a couple of times I had taken a temporary
membership at a gym (usually on a 'free one-month
trial' basis) but that I had never done a full session. The
nearest I had ever got to investing in physical fitness of
any kind was a very basic step machine I had bought
online for £20 but failed to take out of its box. As for
me having a personal trainer, for the last four years my
PT has been Zorro, a dog that insists on dragging me
round various grassy areas at least once a day.

This habit of walking once (often twice) a day, Ash tells me, is probably what has stopped me from atrophying completely, particularly when I was off crutches and recovering from my car accident. I sense from the expression on his face that the adventure that lies ahead of me in the gym is going to be as much of a challenge for Ash as it is for me.

The next day when I arrive for my first session, despite Ash's encouraging enthusiasm, I am terrified. Although weight is not an issue (I weigh something between my winter heavyweight and my summer lightweight), I am nervous of standing on the Body Composition Monitor. This machine measures everything from my BMI (which I now understand to be Body Mass Index), my visceral fat (which is the internal fat around your organs), and my bone and muscle mass. While I am on the machine (that also measures the strength in your arms via grips) the only thing I see is the weight in kilos (which later I translate into 9 stone 6 pounds).

From the expression on Ash's face as he scans the results on the computer, I can tell that my statistics are not that vital.

'Well?' I ask.

'Well,' he echoes, looking from the screen to me. 'There are one or two positives. Your BMI isn't bad and your machine age is lower than your real age.'

'By how much?' I eagerly ask.

'It puts you at fifty-six,' he replies.

This is, to me, an OK-ish result, but Ash seems confident that we can get it lower. And since this is the one challenge in which the aim is actually to become younger — at least in machine years — this number is one I won't forget.

I am wearing the same tracksuit bottoms and T-shirt (washed, of course) that I wore to my first classes of Beginner's Ballroom and the same (now rather tatty) trainers that I stole from my younger daughter. We start on the treadmill and, to my shame, as I have never been on one before, when Ash sets it to my programme (which is really slow) I lose my balance. I think this is the point that the level of fitness I am starting with truly begins to dawn on Ash. The discovery that he needs to teach me to *walk* on a treadmill (let alone run) is clearly a first for him. And, of course, humiliating for me.

Gyms today are so high-tech that they can programme your entire session into your smartphone. Setting this up is part of what the first hour today is about. Everything that Ash takes me through will be recorded on an app on my iPhone, so when I next come I will be able to see what exercise comes next, complete with a demonstration of what to do on each of the machines I use. The theory being that I can come into the gym as often as I like and be able to do my session without a personal trainer like Ash overseeing me.

After ten shaky minutes on the treadmill we go upstairs to the bank of sinister-looking kinesis machines. These machines are one of the main reasons I have never been keen on gyms; to me, they look like high-tech versions of medieval torture devices. Uniformly black, with all sorts of pulleys, hoists, weights and uncomfortable-looking seats, they are designed to force the human body to stretch into unnatural positions (sometimes even upside down). This is made worse, on my first day, by the presence of three or four men contorting themselves (several of them grunting as they do so), displaying the kind of muscles that aren't normally seen outside the pages of publications such as *Men's Health* or *Runners World*.

Ash, who is trying to assess what exactly I need to work on, starts me off on a chest press machine (on the lowest weight). Seated at an angle in which my head and upper body are clamped in an upward position, I pull two weighted wires out as far as my arms can go and then hold them for a couple of seconds before slowly returning to my original position. I repeat fifteen of these movements three times with a short rest break between each set.

'On a scale of one to ten,' Ash asks me, 'how hard was that?'

'A hundred,' I gasp.

'That's good,' he says, with the first of what I come to think of as his winning smiles that stop me from hating him for what he is making me go through.

The really telling test, though, is a deceptively simple exercise on a step-squat machine. Ash asks me to put my right leg on the step and pull my left leg up alongside it — without using my arms to help me — ten times.

This proves almost impossible for me unless I hold on to the handrail on the machine. I then repeat the exercise with my left leg, which is slightly easier, but still requires me to hold on to the safety bar to stop myself from falling over. By now I'm bright red, not so much from exertion as from embarrassment. I don't hear any of the muscle men snigger, but I wouldn't have blamed them if they had.

Ash, who is more accustomed to training thirty- to forty-year-olds than sixty-somethings, turns out to be ridiculously well informed about the physical problems people develop as they age. He decides that the way forward is to begin by working on my balance and posture.

'I think the last government statistics revealed that five thousand older people a year die from injuries caused by a fall,' he says sternly as we move back downstairs. I tell him that I am only too aware of how a simple fall, as I grow older, can impact on my body and affect my life expectancy.

He makes me stand in front of the big mirror at one end of the ground-floor area so that he can demonstrate to me the three points of alignment necessary for good posture. Ash then uses a bar — which looks like a thick six-foot ruler — to show me how I should be standing, indicating the position in which my head, shoulders, mid-back and pelvis should ideally be, with my feet apart but roughly level with my toes 'at eleven and one'. What I realise as I look at my reflection in the mirror is that this is *so* not how I normally stand. My shoulders, in particular, are usually dramatically slumped.

'Most people don't understand how balance works, but with anything — from a building like the Shard to a human body — the centre of gravity has to stay within the base of support,' Ash informs me. 'When you stand properly with those three points of alignment in place and your abdomen braced, the centre of gravity is roughly around your belly button. To remain upright, you have got to stay on your base of support — your feet on the floor — but if your centre of gravity is out of alignment, you are going to fall over.'

'So, in architectural terms, I am the equivalent of the Leaning Tower of Pisa?' I say.

'Exactly! It's surprising you haven't toppled over in the last few years,' Ash adds with another winning smile.

As we age, we have a tendency to lose the correct posture and become round-shouldered, which is an indication that we are leaning forward too much and pushing our centre of gravity out of alignment.

'The other important thing we need to work on is your proprioception — your sense of where your body is in space and time,' Ash says.

There are, he tells me, lots of feedback mechanisms to help us with this — including our eyesight, the receptors in our joints, touch and the fluid in our ears. But as we age, these mechanisms, if they are not used, can decline. That's another reason why we might trip or fall as we get older.

'But don't worry, there are lots of everyday ways of increasing your body awareness that you can do at home, as well as the work we will do here. Try putting your coat on with your eyes shut, or better still, blindly brush your teeth. You'll find it really helps.'

For the first six weeks, he says, we will be concentrating on these two areas in particular – along with starting to build up my core strength to help stabilise another important part of balance: where the bottom of the spine fits into the pelvis.

To complete our hour – which has been more talk than action – Ash suggests we do fifteen minutes on the treadmill.

'A little bit faster, if you can manage that?' he says somewhat harshly, though softened by yet another one of those winning smiles.

I go home feeling a little confused about this introduction to the gym and not at all convinced that I want to go back for the next session (booked in two days' time). There is no doubt that Ash knows what he is doing, but I feel disheartened about the fact that, despite the ballroom dancing and swimming lessons, I will have to work so hard and for so long on my balance and posture, and that I am a long way from getting six-pack abs and pectoral muscles as impressive as Madonna's (well, she's in her sixties too).

The next day I am really, really tempted to cancel Ash, but before I do, I get a message from him saying how well I did in that first session and promising, 'You will feel the difference in less than a month.' It's as though he is psychic. This cheers me enough to make me willing (if not exactly enthusiastic) to go back for at least one more hour in the gym.

Much, much later — when Ash is possibly the most important man in my life — he tells me that right from the start he knew that I was the kind of client that he would have to adopt a 'psychological' approach with to keep them 'on track'. Over the weeks and months that follow, I receive messages of encouragement and lots of links to sites that he thinks will be useful to my research.

He starts that second session by revealing more encouraging (but difficult to understand) developments that will come in the first six weeks.

'What we will be doing with your balance and building your proprioception will be good for your body, but what we are really doing is training your brain. A lot of the developments are going to be in the nervous system. Your brain and your spinal cord are your central nervous system, and the little branches that come off form your peripheral nervous system.' he explains.

I discover that, when I pick up dumb-bells, the trans- mission of this movement starts in the brain, runs down my spinal cord, through all those branches to enter my muscles. This then feeds into a mass of muscle fibres that, for gym virgins like me, won't be working as a unit that fires off with synchronicity — they will be firing off with asynchronicity (which I think means that they are working randomly rather than together).

'So initially, what we are doing is learning to work these muscle fibres together. That will result in big strength gains that help us to refine movement and develop what we call muscle memory,' Ash adds.

This is important for me because in the gym I really am the late developer that my mother insisted I was when I was a child. I learn that the less you work on your muscles, the smaller they will get.

'They will atrophy, but when you work on them and they get bigger it's called hypertrophy. As you age, it's a case of use it or lose it.' (This advice has been thrown at me so much in everything from ballroom dancing to sex that it seems to be the ageing mantra.)

Each session starts on the treadmill with the speed and the gradient steadily going up as the weeks roll on. It is usually during this warm-up that Ash expands on the fascinating facts linked to all the other challenges I am undertaking (it's like walking with Wikipedia). He tells me about Dr Elizabeth Blackburn, who won the Nobel Prize for Medicine for her work with telomeres. These structures, which are found at the ends of chromosomes, can shorten as we get older, contributing to the ageing process.

'It's incredible stuff in that, if we take care of our telomeres by exercising, eating well and doing things like meditation to counteract stress, then we can help stave off the shortening process, and that can delay the move from a health span to a disease span.'

As fascinated by the brain as Professor Simons, Ash's own brain is like a sponge crammed full of knowledge about the power of the brain over the body. He tells me about the Human Calculator, a man called Scott Flansburg, who was born with a rare neurological mutation that enables him to mentally compute advanced maths calculations, codes and patterns. Then there is Wim Hof (a man also much admired by Magic Mike from my meditation classes) who has trained himself to be submerged in ice for two hours without any change to his body temperature (and allegedly climbed Everest barefoot in a pair of shorts).

These conversations with Ash, rather cunningly I eventually decide, usually continue throughout each session and make the time I am strapped into one of those now not-so-sinister kinesis machines seem to go faster. Ash isn't just training me, he is educating me and possibly brainwashing me into believing that I can push a tyre that weighs more than I do across the length of the gym (or at least the two feet that I am capable of pushing it).

In our fourth week I experience a breakthrough and realise that this gym business actually works. We get to the dreaded step-squat machine — the source of much embarrassment during my first session — and I manage to do it without grabbing the safety rail once.

'Hands free!' Ash shouts. 'Now twelve on the other leg!'

A lot of the work he has been doing with me has, like the Aqua-flex classes, been building up my non-dominant side. It turns out, though, that while I am right-handed I have a dominant left leg (this is quite common). Having established this, Ash uses a 2 to 1 ratio on some of the exercises, making my 'bad side' do extra work so that I will become more balanced between my left and my right side.

But while I am feeling the benefits of the strenuous sessions, I know that if it weren't for Ash (and the challenge of this book) I would have dropped out after that first lesson. Although we are now in Week 5 and I am perfectly capable of doing an hour's solo training session with just my iPhone to guide me, I need Ash to keep me going.

I give it a try one day, but without the pushy and persistent Ash to urge me on, I cheat and don't do the things that I don't like. The battle ropes, for example, which weigh heavily when I am trying to keep them moving for thirty seconds. Perhaps this is the bit that is supposed to train my body not so much in space but in *time* — believe me, those thirty seconds can seem like an eternity.

The harder we work, the more I bond with Ash. He has such a positive approach to life and ageing (for someone so young) that I not only trust that whatever horror he puts me through will benefit me, I am also beginning to be motivated to do those things to gain his approval. When we are working on something like my grip, and I am desperately clutching on to a high bar while he times me, what makes me hold on longer than I ever thought would be possible is a need to impress him.

'Nice job, Jane,' he will say, or 'good job' (either way I feel a cross between Jennifer Aniston and Beyoncé).

As we progress — odd as it may sound — I don't see the age gap between us, because he has maturity and wisdom way beyond his years. By which, I hasten to add, I do not mean that I have developed a crush on Ash. I have built up so much respect and rapport with him that I now think of us as friends who are also contemporaries. We talk about everything from politics to parenthood (Ash and his partner Nikki are expecting a baby), and he voluntarily agrees to extend my number of sessions (I have long since used up the ten that were part of my original fee) because he is so determined 'to get results'.

As well as making me work harder physically than I have ever done in my life, he is also making sure I eat regularly because the combination of what I am doing in the gym, in the swimming pool and in my brain-training challenges has somehow had an effect on my appetite, and he thinks I might be losing too much weight.

I remember what Professor Simons said about the brain using more energy than any other human organ; if that's the case, I wonder if I should be increasing the amount I eat. But it's not my healthy, Mediterranean, microbiome-friendly diet (as recommended by Professor Cryan) that's at fault. The problem is, I tend to become so absorbed in what I'm doing that I simply forget to eat.

'What did you have for breakfast this morning?' Ash will demand some days, before admonishing me for coming to the gym on just three cups of coffee. Or he will tell me at the end of a session to go off and make sure I eat a 'proper lunch'.

Ash's brutal brilliance has finally impressed on me the need to hydrate. Although I know (again from my gut regime) that I should drink at least two litres of water a day, I rarely manage to consume more than the sum total of three cups of coffee, two cups of herbal tea and a bedtime glass of water (which is probably no more than one litre).

'Water,' Ash declares, 'is important for just about everything that is going to happen in the body. As little as 2 per cent dehydration can hold back your physical performance and affect how you feel.'

When I say that now I have at least six glasses of tap water a day, he shakes his head and tells me to buy a large 2.2-litre water bottle so that I can properly measure my intake.

At some point in Week 7, Ash has another bright idea that could contribute to my being able to remain physically dextrous for longer.

'I think boxing could give you a real boost,' he says, throwing me a pair of huge gloves and putting pads on his hands.

I am not keen on boxing. Way back — when I was married and my ex-husband was doing some PR for the Lonsdale range of boxing clothing — we were invited to several rather grand boxing events. These often involved us eating a three-course dinner (with copious amounts of wine) at tables placed around the boxing ring while various young hopefuls punched the hell out of each other. We were also once in the front row of a World

Heavyweight Championship fight when a left (or maybe a right) hook resulted in a spray of blood flying through the air and landing perilously close to my seat.

As a result, I have always thought of it as a cruel sport that exposes professional boxers to the possibility of brain damage. And while I knew that Ash wasn't going to land a heavy blow on my hippocampus, I wasn't sure this was the sport for me.

Still, I can't say no to Ash, so I pull the gloves on as tightly as possible (they seem to be one size fits all) and follow instructions as he takes me through 'the old one-two'. With my arms held so that they are protecting my face, and my elbows protecting my body, I jab my left hand into the pad on Ash's right and twist to jab my right hand at his left. After several repetitions (left/right/left/right) that get faster as we go, he moves on to teach me the hook and finally the uppercut (which I struggle with).

'Ash,' I shout after ten minutes of the old one-two. 'I love this, can we do more boxing?'

This is quite a breakthrough because, while I have got used to training on resistance machines and doing things like standing squats, I still, deep down, don't love it. But boxing — well, for some reason I take to it. I'm good enough, he says, to join the Sweatbox class that he runs on Sundays.

'There are two sides to boxing,' Ash tells me. 'There is the physical side of it and the mental side of it, because you have got to have a little bit of intelligence about what you are being asked to do. And it's going to test your power, and power is 70 per cent speed and 30 per cent strength. Then you are going to be using your memory, because you need to remember the routines we are going to perform — there are a lot of different factors but it could be very good for you.'

In Week 10, which is about halfway through my five-month gym challenge — I decide it is time to throw away my tatty T-shirt and tracksuit bottoms and get some 'gym wear'. I don't — as Belle inevitably suggests I should — go to top-of-the-range places such as Sweaty Betty or Lululemon (where leggings can be upwards of around £70) and instead go to Decathlon (where leggings start at £3.49). I buy a black pair for £6.99 and match them with a £4.99 long-sleeved black top. Job done.

It is the first time in my life that I have worn leggings, but then it is the first time in my life that I have attended a boxing class and I don't want to stand out any more than I do (the average age of the boxing class is about thirty-two). If the rest of the amateur boxers that day were surprised to see a woman of my age doing left hooks, it wasn't obvious. And while I was a bit of a lightweight (in terms of power to the punch) they were kind to me, and the young woman I was teamed up with was very patient and encouraging rather than patronising (well, I am a granny).

I do OK in the first half hour of jabbing and hooking, but when it gets to the circuit training side I am, clearly, punching well above my weight. I finish the hour alone on a treadmill.

I am, of course, consistently bottom of the class but I do improve slightly (although one week I nearly get KO'd by a partner who looks delicate but can really pack a punch). I think it is helping with my coordination and my reaction times, and it is definitely helping me to focus and boost my memory. Ash advocates the Spoken Thought system I use in my advanced driving classes (and also used in ballroom) to help me memorise the sequences we are learning. 'Left, right, left, right, hook,' I shout, usually getting to the hook (or the uppercut) a few seconds behind everyone else.

* * *

By my fourth month I am beginning to understand why people can get addicted to exercise. I am not a natural, and on the few occasions when I do train alone I don't push myself in the way I do when I am working with Ash, but I feel better physically, more energetic and so good after every session that I fear that Ash may have succeeded in turning me into a gym bunny. I know that some of these positive feelings are probably caused by the endorphins that my body releases when I exercise, triggering a natural high (often compared to the effect of morphine), but a lot of it, for me, is down to how ridiculously proud (OK, smug) I feel about having stayed the course.

'Tomorrow,' Ash says one day when I am leaving the gym, 'we will get you back on the Body Composition Monitor and see what's changed.'

That night I nervously wonder if the changes I have noticed over the last few months are all in my head, given that I have been on a natural high after every session, and it is the brain that controls so much of what I have been doing. I steel myself for disappointment, recalling Belle's mantra: 'Muscle weighs more than fat'. But I don't think I have imagined this feeling of being, well, leaner and meaner (although I don't have scales at home to put it to the test).

'D-Day,' Ash says when I arrive the next morning.

I take off my trainers and stand nervously barefoot on the machine that will feed back to the computer the new readings on my visceral fat, my BMI and, crucially, my machine age. I grip the handles that measure my arms' strength and wait as the machine does its work.

It takes Ash about five minutes to bring up the original figures and compare them to the new readings.

'Do you want the good news first or the bad news?' he says with an unusually serious face.

'Oh, the good news please, if there is any?' I mutter.

'The good news is that there is absolutely no bad news,' he says triumphantly.

The results on the computer are indecipherable to me, with diagrams showing lines going up and coming down and most of the figures in kg.

I look blankly at Ash.

'Your BMI — which wasn't terrible to begin with — has gone down from 22.3 to 18.6, which is just about perfect. Your muscle mass is up, as is your bone mass.'

None of this means anything to me but Ash seems pleased.

'Anything else?' I ask.

'The machine can't measure everything — I mean, we have improved your posture, and your core strength is obviously so much better. Remember you couldn't push that tyre more than about two feet? The fact you can now push it five times as far proves that,' he goes on.

'But machine proof? Is there anything else I can boast about?' I reply, desperate for approval.

'Your weight has gone down by 11 kilos.'

'What's that in English?'

'You are 8 stone now and you were 9 stone 6 pounds. That's a big loss — maybe slightly too big,' he adds.

Now I know that I shouldn't be thrilled by my weight loss, because it isn't as important as my bone or muscle mass improvements or my shiny new BMI, but I am nonetheless amazed and excited. My life for the last five months has involved so much brain and body work — in the gym and on other challenges — that I haven't had time to think about my appearance. I've been wearing the kind of clothes (chiefly tracksuit bottoms and leggings) that make it difficult to gauge how much weight I might have lost. I totally support the Body Positivity movement and disapprove of the pressure on women to diet to some idealised shape enforced on them by the patriarchy, but I feel that my weight loss has been earned by hard work, and that's the kind of reward that I can legitimately enjoy.

'Perhaps the most impressive result,' Ash carries on, 'is in the visceral fat that builds up around your organs, regardless of how slim you are. Yours has gone down from nine when we started, to four now – and that's brilliant.'

I am positively glowing with pride at this, and desperate to go home and post my results on Instagram (and try on the clothes lurking at the back of my wardrobe that I haven't been able to wear for the last couple of years). I effusively thank Ash, telling him I know I couldn't have made it through five months without him.

'And then there is that other little thing you might really be keen to know,' he says with a particularly winning smile. 'Your *machine age*. If you remember, when we started it was a little under your real age.'

'Fifty-six,' I reply, because of course I remember that number.

'Right then, how old do you think you are in machine years now?' Ash asks.

I look at him nervously because, although none of my other challenges were intended to make me younger, this one was. No matter how good I feel and how improved key things such as my balance and strength are, there will be no denying the number the machine spits out.

'Fifty-five?' I suggest.

'Nowhere near,' he teases. 'Guess again.'

'Up or down?' I ask, somewhat anxiously.

'Down,' he replies.

'Oh, just tell me, Ash. How old I am I?'

'Forty-eight!' he gleefully declares. 'You have managed to turn back the time on your body clock by eight years.'

This is the best news of all as it is proof positive that this challenge has worked.

'That is fantastic! I can't believe it, Ash. Thank you, thank you, thank you' I say while moving towards the door in my eagerness to get back home to write that boasting Instagram post.

'Where do you think you're going?' Ash asks in his stern voice. 'Get back in the gym! This isn't over. This is for the rest of your life.'

I look a little downcast — I hadn't expected to train today — but I know he is right. So I get back on the treadmill, aware that for all the gains — and amazing losses — I have made with Ash in the gym and on the punchbag — I am very much still *a work in progress*.

11

GREY MATTERS

In which my brain is seriously tested . . .

I am ridiculously nervous when I arrive in Cambridge one cool morning at the beginning of June. I am here today to take some tests, and no, I am not hoping to gain a place to study the Recorder at the Faculty of Music, or take a Masters in French at the Faculty of Modern and Medieval Languages.

The tests I will be taking at the BCNI (Behavioural and Clinical Neuroscience Institute) with Professor Jon Simons' PhD student Saana Korkki do not require any qualifications. Which is just as well because I failed the 11+ and only managed to gain six O levels, two CSEs and A levels in English and British Constitution. Hardly enough to get me into one of those obscure degree courses such as Baking Technology Management or Underwater Basket Weaving available (truly) at equally obscure universities, never mind Oxbridge.

What Saana will be testing me on isn't my seven-times table (although, oddly, that does crop up), or my ability to name all the countries in the European Union. She will be testing key parts of my brain that, I am afraid, will expose me as the fraud I have always secretly thought I was (a person of very little brain).

The odd timing of these tests is not entirely my fault. Back in April when I first consulted Professor Simons about this book, he had suggested a before-and-after testing of my cognitive skills. But for various reasons — Cambridge end-of-year exams, May Balls, and Saana's PhD thesis taking up all her time — I was not able to get a date until now. The Professor (who is not here today) is aware that I have already started most of the challenges that he helped me select, but does not think that it will impact too much on the results.

When I arrive at the BCNI, Saana (who I have met briefly on a previous visit) greets me with an encouraging smile and a steadying hand (rather as you would a little old lady, but then to her I am just that).

Very warm and naturally pretty in that uniquely Scandinavian way (Saana is Finnish), she sits me at a desk in the Memory Laboratory and tells me not to worry. In front of me, alongside a glass of water and a pen, is the first test paper.

This turns out to be a version of the MoCA (Montreal Cognitive Assessment), and involves things like drawing a clock with the time set at ten past eleven; identifying obvious wild animals (apart from a trick one-humped dromedary that I nearly named a camel); subtracting from 100 backwards by 7 each time (i.e. 93, 86, 79, and so on). There is also a reaction time test where you have to tap the table every time you hear a particular letter (A) in a long list of letters that Saana, in her gentle, barely accented English, reads out.

I am not at all sure how I am doing (I will not get the results until after I return to be retested), and while it seems quite simple I worry that it is anything but. The dromedary, in particular, has made me fear that there are other dark, twisted tricks I might have missed. I do know, though, that the scoring of the MoCA test is a way of identifying if a person is suffering from MCI (mild cognitive impairment) or Alzheimer's disease, which is, of course, even more of a worry.

Next up is a test of my logical memory, which involves Saana reading a story and then asking me to immediately repeat what I can remember. Since the story is rather like a report from a local newspaper, about a single mother of four children who is mugged and goes to the police who take pity on her and raise the amount of money that was stolen, I should be able to repeat this with a degree of accuracy (I am, after all, a journalist, a profession that purports to make you a *trained observer*).

But when Saana reads the story again I am horrified by how many details I left out. The same happens with the second story and now I am panicking about my hippocampus (or is it my cortex?).

The tests seem to go on forever; there is a drawing challenge (to measure my *visuospatial abilities and memory*) in which I have to copy a strange drawing of what looks like a cross between a very difficult maths diagram and a Star Wars spaceship. Half an hour later, Saana moves me on to two 'trails' — complex versions of the kind of dot-to-dot games I used to love as a child — that will calculate my processing speed and executive function.

But when the trails, which go all the way from A to Z, are connected up, they do not reveal the shape of a little dog or a train, as I had expected — they are totally abstract. At least, I think they are, but then I have always had a problem with those last letters in the alphabet (Q, P, R onwards) and I worry that I have made mistakes and they should have revealed the outline of the *Mona Lisa* or the Houses of Parliament. By now I am feeling frazzled and confused (and I know confusion is not a good sign). This worsens when Saana asks me to redraw the complicated spaceship/maths diagram from memory. It doesn't go well.

Nor does the measuring of my working memory, where I have to repeat increasing sequences of numbers accurately forwards and backwards (never easy for me).

My favourite test is the precision task, which I take on a computer. This measures the accuracy with which I can remember the location and the colour of objects in dozens of different, slightly bizarre scenes that flash across the screen (for example a green chair positioned on top of the Acropolis and a blue pineapple to the left of a desert mountain).

Finally, I have to fill in a questionnaire assessing my 'subjective memory complaints' — rating myself on things like the number of times I mislay things, do I think I'm getting worse, is my memory in general declining?

As soon as Saana says we are finished I find myself haranguing her with questions about how she thinks I did. Didn't she think I was a bit slow on my reactions? Was that dromedary the only trick question? Did my drawing look more like a complicated maths diagram than a spaceship? On and on I go in an embarrassing display of insecurity that is rewarded by an enigmatic smile from Saana (who, I discover later, knew the results then and there).

'Professor Simons will let you know when we have retested you and compared the results,' Saana says, when she finally manages to get me out of the Memory Lab and through the front door. Now where did I park my car, and where are the keys?

* * *

Back home later that day I reflect on how this whole mad challenge came about and how far I have come — and still have to go — to complete it.

I first came across the Professor (who was then Dr Jon) several years ago when I was researching an article about memory for the *Telegraph*. It had been inspired by my concern about how often social occasions (meals out with friends, parties, coffee meet-ups and so on) were becoming dominated not by gossip or politics but by what I termed *Senior Charades*. This was what happened

214

when one or other of us would struggle to recall the name of, say, a famous actor in a recent film and the rest would try to help them remember.

'You know who I mean,' someone will say. 'He was in that film — oh, what was it called? It had something to do with the First World War . . .'

The follow-up would involve a deluge of questions in which the rest of us would, in trying to help out, only add to the confusion of who was 'what's-his-name'.

'Was he the one who married that actress that got an Oscar for that film — I can't remember the name, but she played a man?' is a typical response that will throw the game even wider, adding a 'what's-her-name', plus another film title to recall.

Senior Charades ends, sometimes days later, when one or other of us will send a group message, often in the middle of the night, listing the names none of us could remember. This person is the winner.

Jon Simons was crucial in overseeing this article and explaining that the two most common problems that people encounter as they age — Absentmindedness (losing your car keys and so on) and Blocking (also known as tip-of-the-tongue syndrome) — are entirely normal.

Blocking, which often results in a game of Senior Charades, is when you cannot retrieve information from your brain even though you know it is in there. This happens because in searching for the right name we think of other similar names that are blocking the right one. There is no solution to blocking apart from thinking about something totally different and hoping that at some point that name will come back to you.

I wondered if this problem was linked to our growing dependence on smartphones, and the fact that we are now able to retrieve so much information online that we have lost our ability to retain knowledge. Dr Jon dismissed the idea of the 'Google effect', telling me that every technological advance has prompted concerns that it will be detrimental to our health and well-being. Humanity has always been fearful of technology. When the calculator was invented, for example, it was thought that humans would no longer be able to do mental arithmetic.

The brain, Professor Jon asserted (and he should know), loves to offload some of the demands made on it (it is, after all, incredibly busy). The smartphone, he said, could be regarded as an external extension to our brains that gives us so much more cognitive stimulation than we had fifty years ago in the days of black-and-white television and the Encyclopaedia Britannica.

I questioned whether this was another cause of my tip-of-the-tongue problem. I have been taking in so much information during my life, and particularly since the digital revolution, that maybe it was a simple case of 'memory full'?

And Dr Jon's answer, *truthfully*, is what inspired me to write this book.

'There are around a hundred billion neurons in the human brain and there is no possibility of filling that up in a lifetime,' he said. 'And while the frontal lobe is not going to function at sixty as it did at twenty, there is plenty of space and life left in the brain. You just have to keep on challenging it.'

And, boy, am I doing that . . . .

* * *

In the four months between my two tests, simultan-eously undertaking most of my various challenges, I work harder than I have ever done in my life (OK I did take ten days out to talk French in France). This is not, as you might assume, because I am a stranger to hard work. For a large portion of my life I was a working mother raising three children — my first child arriving in 1980 and my third in 1992 — which was, to say the least, challenging. But what I have done over the months that I have been focused on attempting to future-proof my brain and my body, has involved so much physical and mental exertion that nothing I have done in the past can compare to what I am doing now.

In addition to learning French, life drawing, dancing, music, press-ups and reversing a car, I have also been doing quite a few other things that I hope might help me on my journey to old age. In what downtime I have (about an hour before bedtime at 9 p.m.) I have been doing other cognitive exercises to help me reach my goal. Professor Simons had been sceptical about the benefits of my doing things like Sudoku and Codeword every day (which I do) because, while they are initially a challenge, as you gradually improve to the point where they are easy to complete they cease to bother your brain.

But he did suggest that, in addition to my main challenges, I should increase the number of brain-training games and do them in rotation every evening so that they are continually testing me. The only thing I must not do, he says, is pay for them.

'If they are free and you enjoy them and feel they are challenging you, then they probably are, but don't get caught up on a game that charges you for clues or virtual riches that will aid your progress,' he warns.

I duly download a few free apps that claim to increase my brainpower and boost my memory — One Brain, Word Collect, Memorama, Word Stacks, Elevate and something called Two Dots.

One Brain and Elevate genuinely seem hard and require a great deal of concentration, so they become the least visited of my end-of-a-busy-day games. The ones that involve word-power all seem to have originated in the US and include words that are often more confusing than my French. But once I have worked out that mobiles are cells, expressways are roads, to broil is to grill and an aubergine is an eggplant, there is no challenge whatsoever to Word Stacks or Word Collect.

But Two Dots? Well, I find myself not just challenged, but addicted to this game. At every turn and level (I am currently on 1062 and there is no end in sight) it tests me in a way I think is good for my brain but which, against the Professor's advice, is bad for my bank balance. Desperate to get to the next level, I find myself regularly paying £2.99 to access the 'gold' I have built up so I can buy 'Booster Boxes' and various other items that will help me move forward. I justify this by thinking that anything is worth the possibility of a good score in my second test.

I have also implemented what is known as a 'proactive brain health plan' by taking daily doses of vitamins and supplements that claim to boost brain function (the only supplement I usually take is Vitamin D). I do not tell Professor Jon about this because I know he is sceptical about the need for food supplements if you have a reasonably healthy diet and lifestyle. But I have been recommended (by the husband of a friend who is a brilliant scientist) to take a supplement called Tri-B. There is, apparently, a 'direct correlation between B12 deficiency and poor brain function' and the combination of B6, B12 and folic acid in Tri-B is said to protect both the brain and the heart.

I also take Vitamin C every day because I probably don't eat enough fruit (although I am good with my greens). A 2014 study by the University of Copenhagen concluded that there is 'increasing evidence that Vitamin C is an important redox homeostatic factor in the central nervous system, linking an inadequate dietary supply of Vitamin C to negative effects on cognitive performance'. And who am I to argue with that?

I add to that a daily dose of Vitamin K, the major function of which is to regulate calcium in the bones and the brain (the 2015 Clip Study suggested that increasing the Vitamin K intake in geriatrics resulted in better cognition and behaviour), and a Vitamin E supplement because a deficiency is believed to have a similarly detrimental effect on cognitive performance. There are so many tablets – some of which are so big they are difficult to swallow – that breakfast each day becomes a cup of coffee and a supplement-sandwich.

My proactive brain plan has another downside because I am forced to buy an extra-large seven-day pillbox so I don't forget to take them – and I had hoped to reach my eighties before I needed to do that. I am generally blessed with good health and am not yet in need of statins or Warfarin or any other of the many things that I know people of my age are prescribed, but then I remind myself *these* pills are not drugs, they are vitamins. And if there is a chance that they will work (and there is no guarantee that they will) I am going to keep taking them.

In August, Belle, who is also on the proactive brain plan (what would I do without her?), calls me to say that she has heard that CBD oil does 'marvellous things' to older adults and suggests we add that to our daily intake. Belle and I discover that in the depths of leafy Oxfordshire, not far from where we both live, there is a hemp farm. They describe themselves as a 'group of motivated and inspired folk dedicated to creating hemp products for the benefit of people, the community and the planet'. Since it is so close, Belle and I set out one day to buy some CBD.. I have to say this is one of the most curious and unlikely trips that Belle and I take in the making of this book.

For a start, it is difficult to find. We venture down unmade one-track lanes in the middle of nowhere, and when we think we have arrived all we can see is a rather pretty but seriously run-down cottage. Belle being Belle (braver and more inquisitive than I am), doesn't hesitate to open the unlocked door and enter the building (with me following behind her).

Inside there are about fourteen 'inspired folk' sitting round a table eating bowls of vegan stew. I feel as if I have somehow travelled back in time to the late 1960s, not just because of their long hair, crazy beards, luxuriant moustaches, embroidered waistcoats and flared jeans, but also because the interior of the building is very *Withnail and I.*

I am not quite sure what they made of these two women — Belle, as ever, dressed immaculately — bursting into their lunch, but they gave us one look and asked if we would like some stew.

Belle said later she thought they offered us lunch because they thought we were there on official business from the Inland Revenue, or maybe the police. I did think that was taking it a bit far — we looked as much like undercover cops as they did estate agents. Anyway, it turned out that they had so few drop-in customers that they always gave them a warm welcome (even if they did think they looked a bit like *Cagney and Lacey.*)

Eventually we communicated why we were here (we were nervous because we thought we might be buying something illegal). Could we possibly buy, I said, some CBD oil, because Belle's husband suffered from arthritis and we had heard it was very helpful.

A rather dashing young man got up from the table and said he would take us to the stockroom (an old shipping container) and we could choose whatever we wanted. He was from southern Siberia (where historically hemp grew naturally but is now a banned substance under Russian law), and he spoke English with such a wonderful accent and was so attractive that Belle and I got quite skittish.

Inside the container there were shelves and shelves of products, from the Full Spectrum CBD oil we had come to buy, to hemp skin moisturisers, hemp tea and hemp salad oil. Our Siberian salesman (we couldn't understand his name but thought it was something like Serge) was so persuasive that Belle and I wanted everything. The cheapest item was the tea at £6 and the most expensive the 600 ml CBD oil at £45. Our only worry then was payment — there was no sign of a checkout till in the container — and we knew that we didn't have enough cash.

'Do you take cards?' Belle asked nervously.

We were then led through to the office (a prefabricated cabin) where half a dozen more 'inspired folk' were sitting at computers taking online orders. Siberian Serge produced a hand-held card machine with a very erratic signal that eventually took £118 from each of our debit cards.

That first evening I very carefully followed Serge's warning, and put just two drops of the oil on my tongue and swallowed it back (it tastes horrible) with a nice cup of hemp tea. I don't remember going to bed but I woke up at 11 a.m. the next morning with what felt like a mild hangover.

I must have slept for about thirteen hours when usually I am lucky to get seven.

At 2 p.m. I got a message from Belle saying that Ed (who doesn't actually have arthritis) still hadn't woken up after the cup of hemp tea he drank at 9 p.m. Did I think she should be worried? I replied that I was sure he would be fine but I was concerned about driving — would it be like getting in the car after five gin and tonics (not that I have ever done that).

We both agreed that we wouldn't risk it.

Later that day I called my son Rufus because I knew (from what he hid in his sock drawer from the age of about fifteen) that he was better informed about illegal substances than either Belle or me (yes, I was a liberal parent, but it's all come out OK — he doesn't even smoke now he's in his twenties).

'Look, Ma, what you have bought may be a mild relaxant and will help with things like pain, but it will not make you high. If it helps you sleep, great, but it's not psychoactive, so of course you can drive,' he said, and since he has more than my one O level in biology (he has an A level and a BSc), I believe him.

I was, if I can be truthful, a little disappointed to discover that it wasn't what you might call the *real thing*. But there is a lot of confusion about the CBD that is legal and the CBD that isn't (the stuff that contains 30 per cent THC). THC (which stands for Tetrahydrocannabinol) is the mind-altering ingredient that is a controlled substance under the misuse of drugs act of 1971. The CBD you can buy legally – in vape shops and in sweets, creams and even sexual lubricants online – must adhere to the EU ruling that 'it has been derived from an industrial hemp strain' which contains 0.2 per cent THC.

With no obvious benefits to my brain (apart from sleep, which the brain loves) it probably doesn't contribute much to support me in my challenges. But I have to admit that a dollop of hemp-seed oil in my vinaigrette dressing does perk up salads, and a calming cup of hemp tea, after a hard day spent boxing, practising the recorder, doing my French homework, swimming and studying the Highway Code helps me to wind down.

* * *

I arrive in Cambridge for my retest in early October, feeling more nervous than I had been in June. I am due to meet Saana at 11 a.m. and since she has been so kind (and I am not beyond bribery), I buy her a travel gift set as she is off on holiday tomorrow, having finally finished her thesis.

We hug like friends when I reach the BCNI and I give her my ingratiating gift, which she seems to like. Ten minutes later it's back to business and I am sitting at that desk again with a glass of water, a pen and the first test paper.

I feel much the same as I did four months ago: unsure whether I am doing well or not. I think that my concentration is better − it should be because the message I have got through all my challenges from the gym to the recorder − is to focus, focus, focus.

I believe that I have gained from the work I have done and, overall, I feel happier, more confident and ridiculously energetic (which I put down to that old adage 'the more you do the more you can do'). But whether that improvement will show up in the results is debatable. These good feelings may be due to a sense of achievement (even if I didn't get to *Strictly Come Dancing*, I did perfect the social foxtrot) than to any genuine improvement in the workings of my brain.

This time when the tests end I don't drive Saana mad by questioning her about my performance, because I will be back in couple of weeks for a meeting with Professor Simons in which he will analyse the results. I just wish Sanna a happy holiday and good luck with her thesis, and leave. (Not that she needed luck − Saana won the prestigious Read award for her thesis and is now officially Dr Saana Korkki.)

* * *

It seems a lifetime since I first walked into Professor Jon Simons office a little over four months ago. On the surface, nothing much has changed: his room is still dominated by a large brightly coloured plastic reproduction of the human brain, and the walls are still covered in framed certificates that trace his journey from Cambridge undergraduate to Cambridge professor (with a stint at Harvard along the way). Over his desk, too, there are still lots of pictures of his wife, his children and his dog.

But I feel different. At the outset, when we had gone through all the possible ways in which I could try to boost my brain and body as I grow older, it hadn't occurred to me that doing those things would change me as radically as I think it has.

Before we get to the serious business — a printed breakdown of the results of both my tests — I tell Jon (we are on first-name terms now) about one of the amazing old people that I interviewed in my attempt to understand what it is that keeps certain people sharp, funny and youthful while so many of their contemporaries become depressed, out of touch and negative.

At eighty-seven, Nancy Diamond still works three days a week, albeit voluntarily, at her local theatre and maintains an active social life despite having lost her husband two years ago. Hilarious and articulate, she talked to me for an hour and a half about her attitude to ageing. But it wasn't until I bumped into her, a day or so later, that she revealed what she had decided was the real reason ageing affected people in different ways.

'I know what it is,' she said to me. 'You have to have a project if you are going to keep up with the world and maintain your faculties. And the trouble is that for so many people as they age, the only project they have is their health. It is all they can talk about, all they can think about and it doesn't usually end well.'

I tell Jon that I thought this might be true and that, although Nancy is obviously older than me, I felt that the big project I took on with this book had given me a new enthusiasm for life. Because of that, regardless of the results of the tests, I felt I had learned exactly *How Not to Get Old.*

'That's interesting because, while you have to accept that as you age there will be a gradual physical decline, worrying about that decline and becoming over-sensitive to every ache and pain will put you into a vicious cycle where, if you think you are declining, you will decline.' Jon picks up my results paper and smiles before adding, 'Whereas you, Jane, are in a virtuous cycle.'

Does this mean, I wonder, trying to work out the difference between vicious and virtuous cycles, that my results are positive?

'So is my brain functioning well?' I ask.

'To be honest, when we first started on this I didn't expect any improvement in the time we had. I wouldn't expect any change in cognitive abilities in four months — four months is nothing in terms of the brain. You might expect to see a slight change after a year of working really hard on various cognitive challenges. But your results are quite striking.'

227

He tells me that the results of the MoCA tests had remained the same because my initial score for my age could not be bettered.

'You had the benefit of a good memory to start with, so no change there,' he tells me, which allays my concerns about a score that revealed MCI (Mild Cognitive Impairment) or worse.

The area in which I am most improved — and which Professor Simons is most excited about — is in the tests that measure verbal memory. These were the tasks that involved recalling two different stories immediately after Saana had read them, and again after a twenty-minute delay. There were also points for the number of exact details I remembered and points for the number of questions I answered correctly after a twenty-minute delay. It was these tasks, in particular, that I had thought I had badly let myself down on, yet the results revealed, according to the professor, a dramatic improvement.

'The improvement in your long-term verbal memory is quite significant. Your score for immediate recall went up by eight points — which I would never have expected — and indicates that what you have been doing is definitely working,' Professor Simons continues.

In talking to him over the past few months, while checking out scientific facts for certain of my challenges, I know that Jon is a very cautious man. Every quote he has given me is preceded by a statement such as 'it is thought' or 'there is an idea that', because unless there is irrefutable, scientific proof of whatever I am asking him, he will not count it as fact.

So hearing him being so positive today comes as another surprise. He is unequivocal about my progress and enthusiastic about what it signifies in terms of maintaining and improving cognitive skills when you are in your sixties.

'Another significant improvement is in your digital span – the number of digits in a sequence that you can recall, a measure of your short-term working memory. This is a surprisingly positive result.' He goes on to explain that this indicates improved cognitive flexibility, which is the ability to adapt to change, something that can dramatically decline as we age.

'This is a measure of those executive functions that enable you to hold things in your mind for a period of time and then use that information to make decisions, perform tasks and make plans. All the higher cognitive functions rely on that working memory store. It is one of the really vital parts for maintaining healthy cognitive function. And that result is very interesting.'

When I ask him what he thinks may have caused these unexpected improvements he suggests it is mostly down to the fact that, as I have been learning all these new things – even in the gym and on the dance floor – I have boosted my ability to concentrate and focus.

'Concentration is key. One of the real problems with ageing that makes you more vulnerable to cognitive decline is being able to pay attention without being distracted by other things. So often people say "My memory is getting worse", when it's not their memory, it's their ability to pay attention that is deteriorating,' Jon says.

I tell him how much I initially loathed my gym training, but now I feel it is something that I will do for as long as it is physically possible. He knows, too, how hard I found taking on French again and how testing it was to learn how to play an instrument that I imagined to be child's play.

'What is useful as you age is to motivate yourself to do things that you are not naturally drawn to. It is much easier to not challenge yourself, but doing so can have a strong impact on your cognitive abilities.'

We talk about how useful I have found the 'spoken thought' I first discovered in my advanced driving – and also implemented in other challenges such as boxing – in helping me to focus on what I am doing 'in the moment'.

'Bingo!' Jon shouts. 'Being in the moment, being aware of what is going on around you, focusing and concentration are skills people can definitely improve.'

'At any age?' I ask him.

'I don't see why not,' he replies.

I am now feeling, if not quite 'brilliant', then certainly rather pleased with myself for how well my *How Not to Get Old* experience has worked out. Professor Simons is pleased too, because he feels that the message of the book (in which he has been very much involved) is exactly what it was intended to be and one he is eager to endorse: That your later years can offer you an opportunity to do new things, challenge yourself and enjoy a rich and varied life.

'In some ways it was easier for you to take on these challenges because you have a natural inclincation not to accept the negative aspects of ageing,' he says — referring back, I think, to my history of being totally in denial of the ageing process.

'But even people who don't have that natural sense can see from what you have done that by starting to do this kind of stuff — which is hard work and takes energy and perseverance — they will gradually build up this virtuous cycle. They will realise that they have gone a week without thinking of their aches and pains and the negative sides of ageing. They will be focusing instead on the positives, the improvements and the gains they can still make. Doing these things may not lengthen your life, but the years you do live will be healthy, happy, productive, positive years rather than negative declining years.'

The only problem I have, he tells me as we part, is that I have got to keep on finding new things to challenge me because the brain is easily bored.

'There were two things you refused to take on back in April: maths and anything to do with heights. So to keep your virtuous cycle in motion I suggest at least a GCSE by next summer and maybe Everest?' he says.

I laugh loudly at this, although I have a feeling he is not joking. And as horrendous as the idea of algebra, fractions, calculus and geometry might be — let alone the notion of confronting my fear of heights — I know that I probably need to add them to my ongoing schedule of self-improvement. Because I now know that a life without challenges is no life at all . . .

12

'WHEN SUDDENLY I AM OLD AND START TO WEAR PURPLE'

In which I learn to look in the mirror and make myself visible . . .

I am walking along a crowded pavement in Soho on a wet winter evening when I am suddenly reminded of an ugly childhood memory. I must have been about eight, the youngest of a family group that included my parents, an aunt and uncle and a clutch of cousins on a trip to the theatre. Straggling a little behind the others in the party, I didn't notice them turn into another street until, moments later, I realised they were gone. The way I had felt that night, finding myself lost and alone in a city of bright lights and dark alleys packed with strange giant people who couldn't see me — returned so vividly that I am that child again.

I am so swept up and captured by the memory that for a moment I lose my bearings and I am panicking to find my way back, not to my family, but to the tube station that will take me to safety. I stand on the pavement, trying to remember if I need to go left or right, while people push past me as if I don't exist or, perhaps worse, I do exist but I am worthless, as unimportant in this ghastly landscape as the poor homeless people who are sheltering beneath duvets in pop-up tents.

What is happening to me? I have experienced panic attacks before, but I have never felt as confused as I am now. I cannot move, my heart is racing and I feel dizzy and disorientated. Turning round, I see a couple, about my age, walking towards me. Somehow I manage to get their attention and ask the way to Piccadilly Circus. They point left and as I start walking in that direction I realise I am not that eight-year-old — lost but thankfully found again all those years ago — and the panic slowly subsides.

* * *

On the way home, I began to wonder if my fear and confusion might herald the beginning of what people referred to as a 'second childhood'. Was I approaching Shakespeare's seventh age of man — 'returned to a second stage of helplessness'? A time of my life when I would neither be seen nor heard?

I had, of course, long been aware of the way older people cease to be seen by the wider, younger, world. How many times, on evenings out with female friends of a similar vintage, had we been ignored by restaurant staff who would — when they did finally acknowledge us — place us at a table as far from the front window as possible. I was aware, too, of the way people had begun to talk, well, *down* to me. Adopting the same patronising tone to me that they usually reserved for very young children, people for whom English was not their first language and the hard of hearing. Even my own children had begun to say things to me that suggested they thought I was losing my marbles. 'Have you got your keys, Mum?' or 'Are you sure you should be going out at night on your own?' Those normal day-to-day exchanges with strangers had subtly altered, too, so that the man selling vegetables at the market — who might long ago have called me 'darling' and later 'love' — now just calls me 'dear'.

These changes in the way the world sees you are a fact of older life that you gradually learn to accept. Irritating, but in a way understandable — didn't I, back in my high-viz youth, have a similar response to seniors? It's nature's way.

What was new to me, though, was the feeling of utter vulnerability I had experienced on that Soho street. There had been occasions in my younger life when I had been vulnerable — it was a given during my pregnancies and, more recently, was the overriding emotion after my car accident — but in the past I felt confident that people would view that vulnerability with compassion. Not the disinterest bordering on hostility I sensed during that stressful visit to London.

Which is why, almost at the end of the challenges I took on to age-proof my brain and body, I decided I needed to work on ways that would help me to build up my defences so that I could walk confidently in a world in which ageism is a daily reality.

It was never my intention to venture into the subject of Invisible Woman Syndrome or to start bleating on about wrinkles and age spots, or the way gravity pulls bits of you down until even a good bust bodice (as bras were once known) can't hold you up.

Nor was I going to talk about the hairs on my chinny-chin-chin that I secretly remove every morning with an intimate 'feminine' razor, even though I might do better to invest in a Gillette Mach3 Turbo Men's Razor (which claims to 'Turbo-charge your style' and make 'shaving a high-performance activity'). Looks, and being looked at, had nothing to do with the aim of this book.

Despite my determination to avoid the whole horrid anti-ageing movement that makes sane women in their forties, fifties and sixties imagine that there is some magic cream (or cosmetic procedure) that can make them look twenty years younger, I find I cannot ignore this aspect of the ageing process. By which I don't mean I am about to embark on micro-needling (ouch), or laser resurfacing, or having deoxycholic acid injected into my sagging jawline. I just want to see what I can do to help myself remain visible in a way that is proud and positive, and in no way an attempt to deny who I am or what I have experienced in my life.

Because, apart from a few hairs on my chin, I have always felt that there is a lot that *is* positive about being physically *older*. As problematic as the menopause can be (I was lucky enough to get through that period with nothing worse than hot flushes), it does at least liberate women from all that business that makes men squirm and is, I firmly believe against current thinking, the real *curse* of womanhood.

When I think back to my first period (when I was eleven — the only area in life that I wasn't, as my mother always said, 'a late developer'), I recoil at the memory of the sanitary belt and great big pads that I had to wear under my regulation school knickers. Although Tampax had been available in the UK since 1939 (long before I was born, I hasten to add), it was regarded at my convent school as a product that could only be used by 'married women'. It was, in fact, a secret, sinful box of tampons smuggled into school by my most daring classmate when I was about thirteen that was the closest I ever got to understanding, as I have mentioned before, anything about the vagina. But even then I couldn't, for the life of me, find mine, so it was back to the belt and pad system. But I digress, because one of the greatest blessings of being post-menopausal is waving a grateful goodbye to 'sanitary products' (although I know that these days the cool girls use Moon Cups).

What I am trying to say is that, just as there are things about their bodies that women are urged to keep quiet about when they are young and fertile, so too there are certain things that women in their fifties and sixties tend not to talk about, even with each other.

That, thankfully, doesn't happen with Belle. One of my favourite stories that backs up my belief that a good friend is someone who will tell you the truth no matter how it upsets you, concerns a dog walk that first prompted me to think about the fine line women tread between trying too hard to be visible and not trying at all.

The two of us were emerging from the woods — in pursuit of our dogs — into a rare burst of sunshine when Belle stopped in her tracks staring at me.

'Good Lord, Jane!' she exclaimed in horror, looking at my face now fully illuminated by the sun. 'What is that hanging off your chin?'

Back at Belle's house, sitting in front of her light-up magnifying mirror, I saw what she was talking about. Well, it would be difficult not to, because on the left-hand side of my face, extending at least three inches, was something that looked more like the long leg of a very plump tarantula than a human hair. I was, as you can imagine, shattered by this discovery. How could I have missed this hair, which was long enough to swing around in the wind, when I shaved that morning?

'I'm not sure tweezers will be enough to get rid of that,' she muttered. 'We may need pliers.'

This was a turning point in my relationship with Belle. She is one of those women who always looks perfectly groomed in a way that is totally age appropriate (she has allowed her hair to go a dazzling natural buttery colour and her lovely face is the result of good skincare, not Botox or anything claiming to be 'anti-ageing'). So once she had removed the offending whisker, she went on to talk about the quandary facing the older woman attempting to look modern and relevant without being labelled as a charging cougar or a piece of tough old mutton dressed up like a rack of spring lamb.

'I think that a lot of women believe that there are only two ways a woman can go as she ages. She can follow the lead of the admirably au natural Mary Beard or she can desperately pursue the road followed by Madame Macron and Madonna,' Belle said.

It is, of course, fine to attempt to emulate any of these role models for ageing (being judgemental of another woman's choice is never a good idea). I am a huge fan of Mary Beard (I did rather well in my History O level) and I can see that it would be very liberating to lie back and let nature take its course. In fact, these days letting go and allowing hairs to build up in places they never previously existed (noses! ears! sideburns!) is considered something of a bold feminist statement.

But then I also have a sneaking admiration for Madame Macron, who has an understandable reason to worry about the ageing process since, when she and her husband first met, she was forty and he was just fifteen. Yet maintaining the figure of a pre-pubescent child and the face and hair of a woman fifteen years younger than her sixty-six years must involve so much self-deprivation, discipline, hard work and time that it seems to me to be far too high a price to pay for the privilege of looking good on the world stage. And Madonna? As brilliant at reinventing herself as she might be, and as defiant of the ageing process as she obviously is, there is something rather worrying about her fight to be seen.

Surely, I say to Belle, there is a middle road that women can take as they age? She nods, glances at my reflection, and I realise that of course she is in that middle lane. Her advice, since I don't want to find myself further on the path to 'letting go' but am not prepared go to the extreme lengths necessary to do a Macron or a Madonna, is to have a make-up and beauty update.

I know she is right because the only cream I have used on my skin for the last twenty-odd years is a trusty tub of Astral (about £4 a pot) and my make-up hasn't taken into account the inevitable changes that have occurred to my face during that time. How long before I find myself the object of ridicule as, unable to see my reflection as clearly as I used to, I go out in the midday sun with lipstick smeared on a down-turned mouth, eyebrows crudely drawn in over eyes clogged with mascara, and blobs of blusher unevenly dusted over my cheeks?

For me, as Nigella Lawson admitted when she turned sixty, making up my face before I go out into the world is like donning protective 'armour'. While I am not courageous enough to boldly go out in my naked, natural state, in applying make-up to my face I don't feel that I am betraying the sisterhood or, as my elder daughter says, 'bowing to the Patriarchy'. Because it has nothing to do with trying to recapture the sexual allure of youth − I just want to feel good in the *now*.

I call on the luminous Ruby Hammer (who has an MBE for services to the cosmetic industry) and at fifty-eight looks wonderful without in any way attempting to 'anti-age' herself. She is, I decide, the perfect person to advise me on skincare and ways in which I can, as she puts it, use the positive to blindside the negative.

When we meet, Ruby takes one kind but concerned look at me and asks to see the contents of my handbag. I empty it on to a table between us and squirm a little at the things I hadn't realised were lurking at the bottom.

Ignoring the loose change, dog treats, poo bags, broken sunglasses and the mountain of receipts that are moulded together with chewing gum, she carefully removes my make-up bag and the products that represent my rather basic beauty regime.

Ruby does her best to disguise her reaction to the odd collection of cheap cosmetics, many of them without lids or tops, but I can tell she is shocked. I try to explain that like a lot of women of my age I find the beauty halls in smart department stores and the interior of high street shops or salons specialising in up-market products rather intimidating, and as a result I tend to buy my make-up and beauty products while doing my shopping at Tesco.

I think I see her roll her eyes when she catches sight of the razor I use every morning to mow down the facial hair that might have sprung up overnight (since Belle spotted that thing on my chin, I have been taking extra care). But what worries Ruby most isn't my make-up, it's my skincare (she reassures me that the make-up I bought

241

in the supermarket is fine as it contains the same basic technology as the more expensive brands).

In fact Ruby — make-up artist to an endless number of glamorous A-list actresses and models — says that she spends as much time on preparing their skin as she does on applying make-up. And she does the same for me, sitting me at her workstation in front of a huge mirror that prompts me to pull what my daughters and I call our 'Mirror Face'. This is a bit like applying the most flattering Instagram filters to a picture of yourself, although filters like Clarendon, Gingham, Lark and the rest cannot do as much for your reflection as half-closing your eyes, sucking in your cheeks and tilting your head upwards.

I have been using this pose forever and my girls have picked it up from me, but it was never about trying to look *younger*, it was only used to soften things down and make my face look more like the images of beautiful women that dominate the media and the culture we have lived in for longer than I (or probably my late mother) could/can remember.

The only trouble with pulling a 'Mirror Face' is that as you get older you a) might miss the odd nose or chin hair and b) it does not prepare you for suddenly encountering your reflection in all its natural glory when you unexpectedly come face to face with yourself in a shop mirror and think 'Who on earth is that'? Sitting opposite my naked face while Ruby gently cleanses, exfoliates and massages my skin is a salutary lesson that makes me even more envious of the Mary Beards of this world who are in touch with their reality, in no way vain and probably never receive those short sharp shocks in shops.

Ruby believes that the more time you spend on skin-care as you age, the less you will need make-up. She understands why I have stuck with my basic moisturiser for so long but tells me that, while Astral and other petroleum-based products can be 'great' for areas such as elbows and knees, they are a no-no for the face. I tell Ruby that one of the reasons why I have stuck with my 'old-school' moisturiser is that I am suspicious of the way cosmetic companies blind consumers with science. Since I don't understand what AHAs, Copper Peptide — let alone all those acids (Hyaluronic, Alpha Hydroxy, Kojic etc) — are, it's easier to stick with something simple.

Ruby suggests I ignore the aggressive anti-ageing products and instead invest in a good quality organic range (she is not affiliated to any particular brand).

'I think you will find that creating a ritual of cleansing and nurturing your skin morning and evening won't just enhance your face, it will enhance your life. It's the ultimate me-time for a woman,' she says.

Having spent an hour on prepping my skin — hydrating it with oil, serum and an organic moisturiser — Ruby tells me that the first thing I should do in reappraising my make-up is to 'unemotionally' look at my face and draw up a checklist of the good things that I have going for me, and a list of what is 'not so great'. There is a pause as we both look at the 'empty canvas' in front of us before I start to point out the scar below my right eye, the bags beneath both eyes, the open pores on my nose and, worst of all, the pronounced lines over my top lip that appeared a few years ago that I absolutely *hate*.

'Did you notice what you did there?' Ruby asks me.

'What did I do?' I say, looking blankly back at her.

'You let the negative dominate the positive,' she responds as she studies my face in the mirror to find something for the 'good' list. 'Everyone has something they don't like about themselves, but everyone also has something good they can work on.'

Ruby uses a sponge to apply a thin layer of foundation across my face. Then she uses another, smaller sponge to put concealer on my scar and my eye-bags.

'I am not going to do anything to conceal your lip lines because as long as you have a good base and good lip colour, no one is going to be looking at them apart from you. Everyone else will be looking at your mouth, watching and listening to what is coming out of it,' she tells me.

Ruby then turns her attention to my eyebrows because they 'absolutely define the face', particularly for women who have greying hair.

'This is the one area of the face,' she comments, 'where we lose not gain hair as we age.' (Don't I know it?)

She says I should follow the lead of someone like Helen Mirren (Ruby has worked with her a lot) and use a shade a little darker than my hair, but not too harsh,

244

to highlight my eyebrows. By the time she has artfully shaped and shaded them I can look at myself without putting on my 'mirror face'. It's OK and when she has applied a discreet blusher (above my scar) and lipstick of exactly the right tone, I can see what a difference carefully applied make-up does for my face.

'You need to take a bit more care and time, that's all,' Ruby says as we both look at the finished effect, which is polished but not overdone, giving me what she calls 'a healthy glow that is fresh and modern'.

The key thing, Ruby thinks, for me and indeed any woman who might be fretting over their reflection in their forties, fifties or sixties, is to look at themselves directly and objectively in the face and accept the changes that will inevitably have taken place over the last two, three or four decades.

'Then try to work out what works best for you *now* in a positive way that will be better for your face than Botox or surgery, or any other of the artificial ways in which women are persuaded to believe that they will look younger than they are,' Ruby says, adding that it simply isn't possible to hold back — or even hold still — time for ever.

With a new approach to my make-up and skincare, I already feel so much better and positive about the way I look. I genuinely think that I *have* come to terms with the changes in my face.

Of course it isn't just my face that needs a radical rethink if I want to remain visible as I walk towards the next milestone. I know, too, that I need to have a long hard look at my wardrobe because – like most women – I have filled it with a uniform that I have stuck to for far too long. Belle has been nagging me to 'brighten' up my image for ages because she thinks that my fondness for a monochrome look – black jeans, black or grey tops and the odd white shirt (for special occasions) – is doing me no favours in my attempt to stay 'relevant'.

Belle puts me on to fifty-nine-year-old Helen Venables, managing director of the House of Colour, in the hope that she will persuade me to try something new. Helen's company uses research into colour done in the Bauhaus School of Art and Design in the 1920s, masterminded by the Swiss artist Johannes Itten. In his book, *The Art of Colour*, Itten identifies strategies for successful colour combinations. By following his theories and applying them to our individual skin-tones, Helen believes it is possible to create a co-ordinated wardrobe designed to bring out the best in you, whatever your age and whatever your budget (she confides that when she first discovered the colours that were right for her – in her thirties – she was going through a tough financial time and built up her look in charity shops).

'What we do,' she tells me, 'is analyse what colours work to harmonise with your natural colouring. If you get those colours right – the ones that reflect light up onto your face so that they have a flattering effect that reduces shadows and makes you look fresh and healthy – it transforms you.'

Helen — rather like Ruby — thinks that one of the problems a lot of women face as they age is the inability to adapt to — and maybe to see — the changes in our bodies that will have taken place over the years. After the menopause our metabolism slows, and the shape of our bodies can alter with our weight shifting away from the hips to the waist and the belly.

'One of the reasons a lot of women come to see me is a feeling that they have lost contact with themselves. In our heads we all have this physical image of ourselves — which we develop when we are in our twenties — but which may no longer match with how we actually look in our forties, fifties and sixties. Life changes us, it changes our bodies and, since we are inside those bodies, we don't always notice,' she adds.

It is, in part, this feeling of not knowing who we are that can cause us to lose confidence and feel 'invisible' to the rest of the world. And if you feel invisible you will be invisible. Helen recalls her experience with her late mother when she was in her mid-seventies. Until that time in her life her mother had always been interested in fashion and had never gone out without make-up, but that began to change. Sometimes — when they went on shopping trips together — she would say to Helen that she 'couldn't be bothered' to put on lipstick or take an interest in what she was wearing.

'When we went out on days when she could be bothered, the reaction she got from shop assistants and staff in cafés was completely different from the reaction she

247

got when she couldn't be bothered. If she had lipstick on and looked reasonably smart they would address my mother directly when she bought something, but if she had no make-up on and was wearing her "comfortable" clothes they simply wouldn't see her and talked only to me,' she recalls.

First impressions, whatever our age, are so important. Whether we like it or not, our face and our body become, Helen says, less 'interesting' as we age. Our skin loses vibrancy and our features can fade, and one of the ways in which we can make ourselves more interesting — and noticeable — is to bring back a little bit of the glow of youth by using colours that will help us to stand out.

Helen understands how, for me, black, grey and white have become my non-colours of choice. She suggests that, even if I don't feel able to embrace a complete wardrobe change (which I don't, because the very idea is scary, expensive and wasteful), I could at least use accessories — scarves, jewellery and hats — to add a contrast that could serve to boost my confidence.

'I think that what the right burst of colour can do is brighten you up so that when you meet up with people they don't say "That's a nice jumper" or "Where did you get that dress?" they simply say "*You look well*,"' she says.

If you get that approval, Helen suggests, you will feel good about yourself and it will reinforce the idea in your head that you are 'still me'.

A day or two after I have talked to Helen and have taken her advice (well, I am wearing a brightly coloured cashmere scarf around my neck) I bump into a neighbour I haven't seen for some time. And, in a way that makes me wonder if maybe Helen has tipped her off, she looks at me and says 'You look well, what have you done?'

It shouldn't have come as a surprise to me that a burst of colour can transform a woman and boost her self-esteem. When you think about the older women who stand out in the world — and even in your own friendship groups — they often do so by using colour. The Queen, for example, always wears brightly coloured clothes when she is on public engagements because she needs to be seen. (She was once quoted as saying, 'I can never wear beige because nobody will know who I am.')

There is nothing remotely invisible about designers Zandra Rhodes and Vivienne Westwood — both in their late seventies — or fashion icons Iris Apfel, ninety-six, and Daphne Self, ninety-one. In developing a bold, colourful individual style that is the antithesis of the classic look society prescribes for the older woman, they have held on to their sense of self and demand to be 'seen'.

A friend of mine, a woman who proudly proclaims 'I *am* eighty-seven, you know' every time we meet, reminds me of the famous poem by the late Jenny Joseph, 'Warning':

> *When I am an old woman I shall wear purple*
> *With a red hat which doesn't go, and doesn't suit me.*

This wonderful ode to ageing disgracefully was written by Joseph when she was twenty-nine and was not a self-fulfilling prophecy (she hated purple and regarded 'Warning' — identified by the BBC as Britain's favourite post-war poem — as a 'minor early work'). But it has inspired women all over the world and prompted the creation of the pro-ageing American movement The Red Hat Society. Members of 'the place to have fun after fifty' (you have to be fifty-five to join) wear red hats and purple clothes to their meetings and celebrate — rather than denigrate — old age.

My colourful friend, let's call her Belinda — the only shy, retiring thing about her is her refusal to allow me to use her real name — is never ever seen without her hair freshly set, her make-up expertly applied and a carefully co-ordinated outfit (often topped by a purple trilby). Over tea one afternoon I ask her what she thinks is keeping her so positive, upright and above all *visible* as she hurtles (it's difficult to walk at her pace) towards her nineties.

'Marilyn Monroe once said that a smile is "the best make-up a girl can wear", and that is something that is still true for me,' she says. 'I think the best advice I could give to anyone is to look up, not down, and to smile, because a smile doesn't just naturally lift your face, it is something that is reflected back at you. Who doesn't respond positively — whatever age they are — to a stranger smiling at them in the street?'

Belinda goes on to suggest other — ingeniously simple — ways of maintaining a positive attitude, and your confidence, into *really* old age.

'Grooming is essential,' she informs me. 'One of the signs of impending death in the animal kingdom is when they stop grooming themselves. If you ever catch sight of me without my hair done, my teeth clean and my make-up on, you will know my time has come.'

This makes me laugh but strikes me as a great truth (my fourteen-year-old cat — ninety-seven in dog years — still keeps herself neat and tidy) and maybe this is one of the reasons why I worry so much about 'letting go'. If I stop shaving and allow those hairs on my chin to join up with the ones in my nose, will I be indicating to the world that my time, too, has come?

Back home later that day I find myself following another piece of Belinda's simple but profound advice. I sit down and count — in a numbered list in a notebook — my blessings. These are the things that we often take for granted that make life worth living and make us feel good about ourselves. Belinda's list is a combination of small inconsequential things — singing, snowdrops breaking through the hard winter ground, piping hot baths, roast potatoes, gin and tonic, the History Channel, clean sheets, candles — that she enjoys, as well as the more obvious aids to a happy life (such as friendship and family).

High up on my own list is my dog, Zorro. There are so many ways in which he quietly — and sometimes rather loudly — contributes to my well-being. He forces me out on the darkest of days, he fulfils my overbearing need to feel needed now that my nest is empty, and he connects me to people I might never normally have met (or noticed). It's difficult to think of anything that is as good for your health in what is often referred to as 'later life' as owning a dog.

Even Professor Simons agrees with me on this point. During one of our chats, he tells me that dogs are 'good for the brain' and particularly beneficial for older people. The 'positive feedback' that you get from a dog that follows you with its eyes and is delighted to see you when you get home is, he says, very life-enhancing. Being responsible for feeding and walking that dog helps older people to override the mentality of putting off tasks because they 'can't be bothered'. With a dog, you *have* to get up to feed it and get out to walk it and that – Professor Simons insists – helps to 'break through the barrier of inertia' that can occur in elderly people and enable them to start to build up a 'virtuous cycle'. No one, regardless how old, young or somewhere in the middle they might be, is invisible when accompanied by a dog.

But the most interesting thing about my list, I realise, is how many of my blessings I have discovered in the course of writing this book. Making myself try new things, many of which were totally alien to me, has helped me to break through my 'barrier of inertia' and open up my life. In the course of what has been one of the most daunting, demanding and hard-working years of my life I have gained so much more than improved mental and physical strength.

Who knew that I would find such pleasure and satisfaction in dancing the cha-cha, boxing, playing 'Ode to
Joy' on the recorder (and Two Dots on my smartphone),
drawing and parking my car (as yet, though, I can't add
reciting French verbs or, er, masturbating in front of a
mirror). And who knows what other pleasures I might
discover as I continue to challenge myself in order to
maintain my progress (scuba-diving, base jumping, bee-
keeping, kayaking, juggling?).

Realising how many varied things make me feel good
about myself — and grateful for my growing list of
blessings — is like giving myself therapy and creating
my own anti-depressant. It may not entirely protect me
against having another frightening experience of feeling
lost and invisible when I step out of my comfort zone
(in Zone 1 of the London Underground, for instance)
but it's put me on to a 'virtuous cycle' I intend to keep
travelling on for as long as I can as I learn how *not* to
get old . . .

RESOURCES

Chapter 1

https://www.arnaudslanguagekitchen.com/
Frédéric Bibard, *10 Bed-Time Stories in French and English* (Villiers sur Marne, Talk in French, 2016)

Chapter 2

http://www.ian-waite.com/Events/Classes
https://www.fitstepslife.com/
http://www.cpa.org.uk/information/reviews/shall-we-dance-report.pdf

Chapter 3

https://www.iamroadsmart.com/

Chapter 4

youcanplayit.com, https://www.youtube.com/channel/UCjRO1LHScDOXa-hR8u0ZO2A
Sarah Jeffery, Team Recorder, https://www.youtube.com/user/SarahBlokfluit

Gerald Burakoff and William E. Hettrick, *The Sweet Pipes Recorder Book* (Charles Dumont & Sons, 1982)
Nina Kraus PhD, https://abcnews.go.com/Technology/living-longer-learning-musical-instrument-protects-brain-memory/story?id=15482696

Chapter 5

Dafna Merom et al, 'Swimming and Other Sporting Activities and the Rate of Falls in Older Men: Longitudinal Findings from the Concord Health and Ageing in Men Project', http://www.portis-headopenairpool.org.uk/wp-content/uploads/2014/10/Merom-Am.-J.-Epidemiol.-2014-Swimming-and-falls-in-older-men-1.pdf

Chapter 6

Carol Rinkleib Ellison, *Women's Sexualities: Generations of Women Share intimate Sexual Secrets of Sexual Self-Acceptance* (Oakland, New Harbinger, 2000)
Barry R. Komisaruk and Beverly Whipple, *The Orgasm Answer Guide* (Baltimore, John Hopkins University Press, 2010)
Nan J. Wise and Barry Komisaruk study, 'Brain Activity Unique to Orgasm in Women: An fMRI Analysis'; https://www.newscientist.com/article/2150180-women-dont-need-to-switch-off-to-climax-orgasm-study-shows/
Sh! classes, https://www.sh-womenstore.com/classes.html

Yes intimacy product range, https://www.yesyesyes.org/

Dr David Weeks interviewed in the *Daily Telegraph*,
https://www.telegraph.co.uk/lifestyle/10161279/Sex-is-the-secret-to-looking-younger-claims-researcher.html

Jamie McCartney, *The Great Wall of Vagina*,
https://jamiemccartney.com/portfolio/the-great-wall-of-vagina/

Sophia Wallace, 'A Case for Cliteracy',
TED Talk, https://www.ted.com/talks/sophia_wallace_a_case_for_cliteracy?language=en

Chapter 7

International Zen Association United Kingdom, https://www.izauk.org/

London Buddhist Centre, https://www.lbc.org.uk/

Headspace, https://www.headspace.com/

Be Mindful, https://bemindful.co.uk/

British School of Meditation, https://www.teaching-meditation.co.uk

Sri Chinmoy Centre, https://uk.srichinmoycentre.org

Dominion, https://www.dominionmovement.com/watch

The Game Changers, https://gamechangersmovie.com/

Chapter 8

Jeffrey D. Wammes et al, 'The Drawing Effect:
Evidence for reliable and robust memory benefits
in free recall', https://www.researchgate.net/publication/282658904_The_Drawing_Effect_Evidence_for_Reliable_and_Robust_Memory_Benefits_in_Free_Recall

Eddie Armer, *Beginner's Guide to Life Drawing*
(Westminster, MD, Search Press, 2019)

Love Life Drawing offers free online tutorials on
various aspects of life drawing https://www.lovelife-
drawing.com

The Royal Academy of Arts runs regular four-week
practical evening classes on Drawing the Human
Form (£420) https://www.royalacademy.org.uk/event/
courses-and-classes-drawing-the-human-form-practical

To find if your local life drawing class just Google —
life drawing classes near me

Chapter 9

Macrobiome Purify Programme, https://www.synergy-
worldwide.com/en-gb

Nosh Detox, https://noshdetox.com/

Chapter 12

Ruby Hammer, https://rubyhammer.com/

House of Colour, https://www.houseofcolour.com/

Acknowledgements

Where to start? *So* many people have helped, supported and encouraged me in the making (and doing) of this book that listing everyone is almost a chapter in itself. Firstly, Anna Valentine was the most brilliant editor, constantly guiding and advising me through my year of challenges, and even giving up a lot of her much-earned holiday to remotely edit me from Talum. Thank you, too, to the lovely Lucinda McNeile who seamlessly tidied up my words, and to the team at Orion/Trapeze, Virginia Woolstencroft and Helena Fouracre.

Huge thanks to the effervescent Luigi Bonomi and to Hannah Schofield at LBA Books for all they contributed.

Then, of course, enormous gratitude must go to Belle (real name Annie T. Simons) who accompanied me through so much of *How Not to Get Old* and was my tireless, much-loved cheerleader. How would I have achieved anything, either, without the help of Jon Simons, Professor of Cognitive Neuroscience at the Behavioural and Clinical Neuroscience Unit at Cambridge University who guided me from the initial idea to the final manuscript of this book?

Merci! to the wonderful Arnaud Barge, still teaching me French, and to the inspirational Ash (real name Ashley Lutchmunsing) who daily monitors my star jumps. Praise, too, for (Dr) Des McDermott for teaching me to parallel park, and the magnificent Dee Keane for encouraging me to swim underwater.

I would also like to thank Ian Waite, Mick McNicholas, Mike Newell, Sara Jeffrey, Ruby Hammer, Helen Venables and Wendy Carrig (who took the ridiculously flattering cover photograph).

Thanks to the friends who inspired me along the way — Liv O'Hanlon, Sue Ryan, Annie Chapman, Christine Priestley, Charlie Howard and Jane Trotman.

Finally, my love and thanks to my three wonderful grown-up children: Bryony, Naomi and Rufus who patiently put up with their embarrassing old Mum.

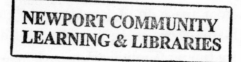

CREDITS

Trapeze would like to thank everyone at Orion who worked on the publication of *How Not to Get Old*.

Agent
Luigi Bonomi

Editor
Anna Valentine

Copy-editor
Anne O'Brien

Proofreader
Kati Nicholl

Editorial Management
Lucinda McNeile
Charlie Panayiotou
Jane Hughes
Alice Davis
Claire Boyle

Audio
Paul Stark
Amber Bates

Contracts
Anne Goddard
Paul Bulos
Jake Alderson

Design
Loulou Clark
Rachael Lancaster
Lucie Stericker
Joanna Ridley
Nick May
Clare Sivell
Helen Ewing

Finance
Jennifer Muchan
Jasdip Nandra
Rabale Mustafa
Elizabeth Beaumont
Sue Baker
Tom Costello

261

Marketing
Lucy Cameron

Production
Katie Horrocks
Fiona McIntosh

Publicity
Virginia Woolstencroft

Sales
Laura Fletcher
Victoria Laws
Esther Waters
Lucy Brem
Frances Doyle
Ben Goddard
Georgina Cutler
Jack Hallam
Ellie Kyrke-Smith
Inês Figuiera
Barbara Ronan
Andrew Hally
Dominic Smith
Deborah Deyong
Lauren Buck
Maggy Park
Linda McGregor

Sinead White
Jemimah James
Rachel Jones
Jack Dennison
Nigel Andrews
Ian Williamson
Julia Benson
Declan Kyle
Robert Mackenzie
Sinead White
Imogen Clarke
Megan Smith
Charlotte Clay
Rebecca Cobbold

Operations
Jo Jacobs
Sharon Willis
Lisa Pryde
Lucy Brem

Rights
Susan Howe
Richard King
Krystyna Kujawinska
Jessica Purdue
Louise Henderson